Praise for *Depression Hates a Moving Target*

"Nita Sweeney's vibrant memoir, *Depression Hates a Moving Target*, not only captures the runner's mind, but shows how practice—whether in running, writing, or meditation—and finding a community can transform a life. Sweeney charts the ups and downs of her journey with searing and refreshing honesty. Her story will resonate with anyone looking for a way out of darkness."

—Natalie Goldberg, bestselling author of *Writing Down the Bones* and *Let the Whole Thundering World Come Home*

"Nita Sweeney's *Depression Hates a Moving Target* is a gallant new memoir about persistence in the face of long odds. If you have an interest in long-distance running, this book has you covered. Dogs? Ditto. A love story? Absolutely! Nita Sweeney not only found a way to survive crippling depression, she created a way to thrive. The love of a good man, the love of a good dog, the love of running, and above all the love of oneself. Come along on this inspiring journey. It goes the distance and then some."

—Lee Martin, author of Pulitzer Prize finalist *The Bright Forever*

"Funny, poignant, touching and inspiring... Nita Sweeney's tale of finding the strength to do what seemed impossible should encourage all of us to get up off that couch and do something to make our lives better! Nita Sweeney is a terrific writer, and her story is irresistible."

—Sean W. Murphy, National Endowment for the Arts Fellow in Creative Writing, author of Hemingway Award-winning novel *The Hope Valley Hubcap King* and *The Time of New Weather*

D0492408

"When we first meet her, Nita Sweeney is overweight, depressed, nearly suicidal. She has run a bit in the past, but things always crashed down around her. This time she sets out again, afraid to tell her friends (because who wants to fail in their friends' eyes?), assisted only by one of those plastic kitchen timers and a dog, Morgan, who walks faster than Nita runs. The voice in her head says, 'You can't do this,' to which Nita replies, 'But I am doing it. Please shut up.' Runners like Nita Sweeney don't win fame and glory, but there are far more of them than there are Olympians. And their stories are just as inspirational. Yes, Sweeney somehow works up to the marathon distance, but it sure doesn't come easy. It takes everything she's got, especially when dark clouds gather overhead. And everything a husband, sister, and great friends can provide. Plus, one more thing, Morgan, the dog. He's as good a coach and training partner as any runner has ever had."

—Amby Burfoot, winner, 1968 Boston Marathon, author of *Run Forever, First Ladies of Running,* and *The Runner's Guide to the Meaning of Life*

"Nita Sweeney's courage and grit shine through her candid memoir of 'running out' depression. This book has the power to inspire countless others as they pace themselves to mental health."

—Aimee Liu, author of *Gaining: The Truth About Life After Eating Disorders*

"Running isn't about how far you go but how far you've come. Nita had to overcome many obstacles to make it to the start line. The finish line was her celebration. Nita used running to gain insight into herself and the world around her, making the human condition more tolerable."

—Bart Yasso, retired *Runner's World* Chief Running Officer, member, RRCA Distance Running Hall of Fame and Running USA Hall of Champions

"Inspiration comes in many forms, and from all sorts of people. Nita's story, told in an open, honest way, will pull at your heartstrings, and hopefully will get you pulling on your shoestrings and following in her footsteps, whether you walk, jog or run!"

—**Darris Blackford, finisher, Badwater 135 Ultramarathon and two-hundred-plus other marathons; Race Director, Nationwide Children's Hospital Columbus Marathon and Half Marathon.**

"Finally, a running memoir for the rest of us. Nita Sweeney's *Depression Hates a Moving Target* is inspiring, moving, and very funny. Her journey is both heroic and deeply human. You don't need a dog or a high-priced pair of running shoes to enjoy this book (but you may end up acquiring them after you finish)."

—**Robert Wilder, author of *Nickel* and *Daddy Needs a Drink***

"Nita Sweeney's *Depression Hates a Moving Target: How Running with My Dog Brought Me Back from the Brink* is compelling. The memoir had me in tears at times, and rejoicing at others. The book (and Nita's life) is a roller-coaster ride, one of the big ones at the super amusement parks, not the teeny ones from our childhood. Wow! The memoir brought back memories of bad form, struggling to make the distance, and that blackout for the last five miles of a first marathon. Well-written, the book is evocative, engaging, inspirational, and compulsive reading. I could not put it down. And what an amazing journey! Nita's strength shines through, as does her struggle and humanity."

—**Paul Nash, ultramarathoner, two-time Comrades Marathon Finisher, Two Oceans Finisher, Boston Qualifier**

"Thrillingly good—an acutely observed memoir that reads like a well-plotted novel. At times funny, gut-wrenching, and frequently both. Nita mesmerizes with tales of the unique life hacks and circuitous corrections she used to cope and triumph. Vibrant, heartfelt, weird, and wonderful, *Depression Hates a Moving Target* will inspire readers to push through challenges to make what seems impossible real."

—Lisa Haneberg, writing coach, author of the novel *Toxic Octopus,* and author of more than a dozen nonfiction books including *High-Impact Middle Management*

"If it isn't hard enough to get out the door and exercise, tack on some serious, chronic depression and see what happens! Nita Sweeney's *Depression Hates a Moving Target* is a poignant tale of one woman's triumphant efforts—first small and then epic—to climb her way back to some kind of life worth living. The book is beautifully well written. Nita's narrative is not just about her, but about the people around her, and soon you begin to care deeply about Nita, her family, and of course her dog. As she trains and runs with Fleet Feet Sports in Columbus, Ohio, pushing through the social anxiety many older runners may feel around younger, thinner, fitter women runners, she finds her group, sticks to a training schedule, and soon, to her own amazement, is exercising nearly every day. Nita's careful to note that running is not a substitute for treatment such as medication and therapy for her mental health conditions. It's just one more tool in the toolbox to help her cope and feel hopeful in spite of everything else. If you're stuck on the couch and doubting whether you could ever enjoy exercising, even if you know it would be good for you, you'll be inspired by Nita's story and leash up your own dog, if you have one, and lace your sneakers to head out the door for a walk or run. And maybe grab a kitchen timer on your way out!"

—Carolee Belkin Walker, author of *Getting My Bounce Back: How I Got Fit, Healthier, and Happier (And You Can, Too)*

"This inspiring and warm-hearted memoir proves that no dream is beyond our reach if we just take one step at a time. I cheered for Nita Sweeney as she described with unflinching honesty her transformation from depressive couch potato to marathon runner, and I laughed out loud at her self-deprecating humor and her conversations with Morgan the dog, her trusty sidekick on the running trail."

—Tania Casselle, award-winning writer and journalist, author of
Insider's Guide to Albuquerque

"Nita's story is a gift, a reminder that you can return to something you used to enjoy. You start with a single step. Even if it means running with a kitchen timer on a secluded street in the neighborhood. Even if it means telling your brain to stop saying 'You're old and fat.' Even if it means that you have to continually fight to get up and just do. Reading Nita's story continuously reminded me of my own journey. Even though our goals are different (because, let's admit it, running a marathon is not one of my goals), her story inspires us to appreciate the small victories along the way to the big goal. Through her grief and loss of loved ones, Nita kept running. Through her fears and daily problems, Nita kept running. Through the health problems and reminders of the past, Nita kept running. The journey continues, teaching us something new each day we attempt to reach the big goal. I can keep running."

—Suzanna Anderson, Editor of *The Magnolia Review*

Depression
Hates a
Moving Target

Depression Hates a Moving Target

How Running with My Dog Brought

Me Back from the Brink

Nita Sweeney

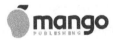

Mango Publishing
CORAL GABLES

Copyright © 2019 by Nita Sweeney

Published by Mango Publishing Group, a division of Mango Media Inc.

Cover and Layout Design: Jermaine Lau

For permission requests, please contact the publisher at:

Mango Publishing Group
2850 Douglas Road, 2nd Floor
Coral Gables, FL 33134 USA
info@mango.bz

For special orders, quantity sales, course adoptions and corporate sales, please email the publisher at sales@mango.bz. For trade and wholesale sales, please contact Ingram Publisher Services at customer.service@ ingramcontent.com or +1.800.509.4887.

Depression Hates a Moving Target: How Running with My Dog Brought Me Back from the Brink

Library of Congress Cataloging
ISBN: (p) 978-1-64250-013-4 (e) 978-1-64250-014-1

Library of Congress Control Number: 2019935676

BISAC category code: SEL011000 SELF-HELP / Mood Disorders / Depression

Printed in the United States of America

For Ed, my husband, best friend, and confidant.

Author's Note

In writing this book, I used my journals and running logs to refresh my recollection of people, places, conversations, and events. I also researched facts and talked to some individuals who appear in the book. As for my opinions, they are my own. I wrote about what worked for me. This book is not intended as a substitute for medical advice on any issue, physical or psychological. As the members of the Dead Runners Society say, "Your mileage may vary."

Table of Contents

Prologue

My mind was trying to kill me again.

"Who do you think you are?" it growled as I squatted in a green porta potty four and a half miles into the Columbus Marathon. The sun shining on the white top bathed me in gray light.

The running partners I'd begun the race with that morning, and trained with for the past four months, had gone ahead without me. They would have stayed. I'd spent a mile convincing them to leave after I could no longer ignore my bowels.

Alone in the fiberglass cubicle, trying to avoid sitting down, I shivered with loneliness as I finished my task.

Mom. Dad. Jamey. All dead.

My ever-faithful husband, my sister, and friends, all still very much alive, were on the course, but miles away. Even the dog, my other regular running companion, was absent—at home—probably asleep.

This left me in treacherous company—with only my mind— forever critical.

Someone in the line outside knocked. I would have to carry my heavy heart across the pavement solo.

"I'm a runner," I whispered to my mind. Then I pulled up my panties, opened the door, and ran.

CHAPTER 1

Off the Sofa and into the Ravine

Five months before my forty-ninth birthday, I slouched on the sofa in my pajamas, squinting at my laptop screen. A high school friend's social media post read, "Call me crazy, but the running is getting to be fun!"

I remembered Kim riding horses in high school, but neither of us had been athletes then, and we certainly weren't now.

I read on. She had begun an interval training plan to run three times a week. The website suggested alternating sixty seconds of jogging with ninety seconds of walking for a total of twenty minutes. Sixty seconds sounded almost possible.

But depression clung to me like a shroud. It was noon on a weekday. As usual, I'd just gotten up and hadn't showered in days. The simple act of walking Morgan, our yellow Labrador, around the block often proved too difficult.

A few minutes into browsing Kim's interval running schedule, an extra-long burst of hiccups reduced me to sobs. I cried until they passed, closed the laptop, and went back to bed.

Still, her running posts nestled like seeds in the back of my consciousness. Later that week, Kim posted, "Week one finished!" Infected by her glee, I remembered the pleasure I'd had when I'd run short distances decades before. A seed sprouted.

Around the same time, Fiona, a writer friend from London, also took up running. She loved buying "trainers" (sneakers). Her emails reminded me of my first trip to a running store, decades earlier, when I'd scoffed at the price tags to hide being intimidated by the options. Fiona also talked about how running felt and the glow after. She is younger than me, but she's not a youngster. The seed grew.

***

Shortly before I saw Kim's post, I'd begun to have a recurring dream. My body gently rocked as I floated down the road through Griggs Reservoir, a wooded park along the Scioto River, near our central Ohio home. My arms, bent at the elbows, swung by my sides. A breeze grazed my face. It felt like flying. The rhythm lulled me back to sleep when I woke from nightmares. There was no anxiety. I wasn't breathing heavily. Relaxed and happy, I was just moving through the bright green world. I was dreaming of running.

***

One March weekday, inspired by the daffodils bursting through the soil of the winter flowerbeds, I returned to the running website. "This might kill you," came the familiar voice in my head. I recalled Kim and Fiona's smiles. Sixty seconds of jogging hadn't killed them.

A wise part of my mind thought exercise might energize me, while a deep animal instinct tried to protect me by scoffing. "You're old and fat. People will make fun of you and you'll die of heart failure." Most people have these competing voices. Mine are just louder.

Drawing strength from the flying and floating sensations of my dreams, I wrestled tube socks over my flabby calves, sweatpants across my wide hips, a long-sleeved T-shirt and hoodie over my thick belly, and a pair of trail shoes, the closest thing to running shoes I owned, onto my swollen feet. Ed, my husband, was at work, so he didn't see my unwieldy outfit.

Morgan circled and nearly knocked me down when I opened the closet where we kept his leash. I would need his support.

I picked up a digital kitchen timer and went outside.

Most of the residents of our maple and sycamore-filled residential neighborhood were at school or work. Even if they were home, they probably weren't looking out the windows of their 1950s ranch houses.

Still, I imagined the neighbors not only watching, but laughing if they saw me try to run. I steered the dog toward Donna Ravine, a secluded street down a hill along a creek, where the houses sit far back on wooded lots.

***

Once I felt safely hidden, I set the timer for sixty seconds and bounced tentatively in my trail shoes.

The small white timer in my sweaty hand was a welcome friend. It had carried me through years of mindfulness meditation periods and decades of the ten-minute "writing practices" I'd learned from author Natalie Goldberg. Perhaps it would serve me well again.

Morgan sniffed, peed on the newly sprouted leaves of a shrub, then stared into the distance.

"This is gonna hurt," I told him.

My mind had replaced the floating feeling of my dreams with a movie montage. First, a day nearly two decades before when I'd pushed myself around an indoor track, gasping dusty air. Then another day when, bone tired from long hours practicing law, I'd cut a run short because I couldn't make it up one more hill. And finally, one day, my mind decided I was through.

The dog stared up at me. He had no fear.

"What do you think, Pink?" I asked, referring to the pink tinge of his almost brown nose.

He cocked his head and perked his copper-colored ears.

I hit the timer button and began to jog.

It hurt.

Pain spread through my chest as my boobs bounced ferociously in my ancient sports bra. Due in part to medications, a healthy portion of the weight I'd gained in the past sixteen years was in my breasts. I slowed and bent my knees. This reduced the bouncing and hurt less. I wondered if it was also easier on my joints. I would later learn this was true.

In sixty seconds, the timer went off.

When I yelled, "We did it!" Morgan looked confused. I'd been jogging so slowly he hadn't needed to break stride.

I didn't care. I tasted victory. Pleasant memories from decades past surfaced. Running in the rain, happy and soaked, feeling tough as I plowed through puddles. Outrunning younger men. Feeling strong, young, and pretty.

But as we walk/jogged our way out of the ravine to where the homes sit closer to the road, these images of running glory faded. The windows stared at me. I turned around and jogged back down the hill, out of view.

In the safe, secluded ravine, I alternated walking and jogging for twenty minutes. The dog continued to walk no matter how fast I thought I was going. When I finished, I breathed heavily, while he barely panted. No matter. I was sweating. It had been a long time since I'd sweated from exertion and the sweat made me smile.

The walk home felt like floating. I glowed inside from pride and outside from sweat. I had run. And, I couldn't wait to run again. But first, I needed a nap. When I lay down, I dreamed I was flying.

That evening, I emptied a can of green beans into a saucepan while Ed sautéed chicken. I said nothing about my accomplishment. I'd given up running so many times before. When the food was ready, I ate hungrily as we talked about whether to buy dogwood trees for the front yard.

I spent the next day at a coffeehouse working on the novel I was revising. As I rewrote the same sentence, I renewed my resolve not to tell anyone. That night, when I talked on the phone to my sister Amy, I did not tell her either. Besides Ed, she's my closest confidante. Amy is eight years older than me, and my brother, Jim, is two years older than her. They parented me as much as our mother and father did. I told none of them, because I didn't want them to get their hopes up that I would lose more weight, have more energy, keep track of stuff I kept losing, be able to shop for groceries, remember where I was going when I left the house, or care more about anything. I didn't want to let them down if I failed. I also didn't want anyone to discourage me. It never occurred to me that people might cheer.

In truth, I was guarding my own hopes. If I told no one, it wasn't real. This small victory was my imaginary friend. I could cling to it regardless of where the jogging thing went.

***

After my first successful day of jogging, I waited the suggested two days to pull on my trail shoes. I had long since discarded my old running shoes. I owned Velcro tennis shoes, but didn't want to feel like the middle-aged grandmother I am, so I chose shoes that lace up. Despite my graying temples and upper lip lines, I have the heart of a curly-haired three-year-old. Perhaps running was a way back to her.

The sweatpants had been too bulky, so I dug out the bell-bottom tights I used to wear at Nia, a dance class I'd taken in a previous attempt to lose weight and reduce mood swings. With spandex containing my thighs, at least my bottom half felt athletic. But no amount of ab work can tone away poor posture. My slouch embarrassed me even when I was at my smallest adult weight. I covered my midsection with two layers.

When I accidentally hit the button on the timer, Morgan, who'd been sleeping calmly at the opposite end of the house, sprinted over. Grateful for his company, I leashed him and headed back to the secluded ravine.

As we walked, I remembered my breathless gasps as I'd pounded my way around the track at a health club twenty years before. I stopped and looked down at the timer in my hand. That first jog had been a fluke. I'd never make it out of the ravine. Running was for younger, skinnier people.

As if they'd heard me, Kim and Fiona's comments filled my head and my eyes dampened.

I'd stood in one spot long enough that the dog had wandered away to sniff a purple crocus. I pulled him back and got the stink eye.

"I need you," I said. He rolled his eyes as if to say, "I'm waiting!"

We began, but I started too fast and was bouncing. Instinctively, I knew every part of my body should move forward rather than up and down. I tried to keep my feet and center of gravity close to the ground. This was more comfortable. Sixty seconds was almost enjoyable. The dog walking beside me paid no attention. When the timer went off, my breath was quick, but not so rapid that I thought I might have a heart attack. I imagined myself running more.

***

At the end of the next run interval, I pulled the dog up short. We'd come to the top of the ravine hill. The gaping windows of the houses on the street glared at us. The dog faced me, then sat.

Part of me knew no one was watching. What ought to have been an easy decision was, for me, an epic struggle. I've heard minds like mine described as a ghetto. You shouldn't spend much time there without backup.

From decades of facing various phobias, I knew that whatever I ran from would trap me, constricting my world. If I stayed in the ravine, I might never go beyond week one of the training plan. I wanted to give running a decent shot. The dog stood and turned to face the open neighborhood.

Instead of heading back, we jogged up the street where, if they had been looking, which they probably weren't, my neighbors might see me waddling slowly enough that the dog didn't notice I'd changed my gait. I focused straight ahead so I wouldn't see the neighbors not staring as we passed house after house. "Look at me jogging in public!" my inner three-year-old cried. When the timer signaled our walk break, you'd have thought I'd run a marathon. Breathing hard was fabulous. I held my head high. The dog sniffed a signpost and peed on it.

***

Morgan and I completed the three identical workouts of week one. I wasn't as breathless or tired as I'd been the first two days and considered a nap, but didn't need one.

Napping is a barometer of my mental health. My alcoholic mother was a well-practiced napper, a skill I didn't appreciate until my own depression made it a necessity. When I don't nap, I feel less like a drain on society, since at least I'm awake during daylight hours. I'm not usually physically tired. Rather, daily living exhausts me mentally. Worn down by the fight, when the bed calls, I succumb. While my newfound jogging wouldn't have been a huge challenge by most athletes' standards, I counted a victory when, after this first week, I didn't nap.

***

The second week of the training plan increased the "jogging" from sixty seconds to ninety. Since it was gradual, the increase didn't freak me out.

Real runners might take offense at the plan's use of the word "jogging." Not me. "Jogging" was still faster than lying in bed. Plus, if it had said "running," I'd have imagined sprinting and been intimidated. "Running" reminded me of my previous failed attempts. Jogging implied ease and comfort. My couch-potato body and easily frightened brain liked this. "Just a little jog," I told the dog. No need to panic.

We went for our little jog. Like the first week, I thought of the people in their houses possibly laughing at me in my oversized T-shirt and spandex bell bottoms with the dog walking beside. But I pushed the thoughts away and continued, challenged, but successful.

After the first day of week two, I again needed a nap, but on the second day, I didn't. I went home, changed into regular clothes, since I barely broke a sweat, and went on with my day. After the third day, I had more energy. This surprised me. In my previous running days, when I ran before work, I'd have to close my office door and take a power nap before starting the day. What I was doing now seemed completely different. I was still napping on the days when I wasn't exercising, but it was an improvement. My friend Kim had called running "fun." I almost agreed with her.

Despite my success, I still had to talk myself into every workout. Feelings of dread plagued me, while a tyrannical inner voice mocked. "Look at you in your 'workout' clothes, pretending to exercise. Save yourself the embarrassment and play computer solitaire instead." Rejecting those voices and working out anyway renewed my sense of self-esteem and accomplishment. I almost enjoyed it, especially once we had finished.

CHAPTER 2

Private Runner

After I completed week two, I was ready to tell Ed. By then, he and I had been married for almost two decades. Ed, my best friend and confidant, has the brains and motivation. I have the harebrained ideas. When I decided we should move to New Mexico so I could study writing with Natalie Goldberg, Ed eagerly accepted the challenge. When I wanted to turn our basement into a meditation studio, Ed moved the furniture. And when I wound up in the psych ward on the weekend after our first wedding anniversary, a surprise that might have made other men flee, Ed didn't falter. Through pastels, piano lessons, dance classes, dog training, and weird diets, not to mention enough types of therapy to fill an encyclopedia, Ed remained by my side. Still, I feared telling him because of how much I value his opinion.

He and I sat in our galley kitchen, at the rectangular table, eating the Italian sausage and lentils he'd prepared. Thankfully, he loves to cook. If he didn't, we'd starve. I open cans, operate the microwave, and wash the dishes, but because of my inability to focus, when I cook, the fire alarm usually goes off. Once, I even warped a pressure cooker. Ed prefers I not cook so I don't ruin his expensive pans.

His long-sleeved, red button-down matched his brown and red oxfords. The red collar against his clear, fair skin made it glow. He'd rolled the shirt cuffs up, exposing his muscular forearms, which flexed when he reached for his fork.

I looked out the picture window to our tree-lined street where I'd been secretly jogging. Our oak had begun to bud, pushing the previous year's leaves onto the still brown grass.

"I started running again," I said.

As Ed knew, I'd run before, but never stuck with it. Once in high school. Once in college. Once during the late 1980s and early 1990s, and for a few short weeks in 2008. In high school, I ran to lose weight. None of my high school pictures show me even slightly overweight, but I thought of myself as enormous. I pounded down the road thinking, *This sucks.* Band practice and daydreaming about boys were more important.

In college, I ran with my friend Priscilla up and down the brick streets of Athens, Ohio. The Appalachian hills were daunting. I gasped for air and didn't love it. I hated my body for not being able to travel along the ground swiftly. When a bout of suffocating depression struck, I abandoned everything not related to academics. I graduated and went on to law school, but stopped running.

In the late 1980s, while practicing law for a small firm, I sat at a desk all day, feeling fat and disillusioned. I decided to run up the hill near my house. I made it halfway before I needed to walk, but when I reached the top, I ran again. This time, I felt the joy and kept running for a few years. I ran on the track at the health club and, with our two dogs, through our suburban neighborhood, dodging neighbors' golden retrievers and small children.

When Ed and I got together, we moved closer to my office, and I ran around a nearby park. I lost weight and felt fit. I also lifted weights and, for a time, thought of myself as healthy. But some internal switch flipped. I was not yet diagnosed as bipolar but was likely hypomanic. When I grew dangerously thin, a therapist suggested treatment for eating disorders. I continued running, but with no joy, and I dieted compulsively. Running swung from something I enjoyed to a dangerous obsession. Eventually, the flat, numb, hollowed-out emptiness of depression took over. I had never expected to run again, and I doubt Ed thought I would either.

I turned to face him. His bright blue eyes were soft and hopeful. Too hopeful.

"Not far and not fast!" I added.

I told him about Kim and Fiona, then explained the kitchen timer and how the dog and I alternated jogging and walking.

He set down his fork and clasped a handful of his more-salt-than-pepper hair the way he does when he's thinking. This tilted his head and made his jaw look even more square.

"Do you have a goal?" he asked.

I shrugged. "It just feels good to be moving."

He released the handful of hair, picked up his fork, and continued eating.

"Don't be a runner," he said between bites. "Be an interval trainer."

Ed's humor tends to be dry, so I waited to make sure he wasn't joking. He wasn't. He'd recently read several articles about the effectiveness of interval training and the importance of starting slowly.

I smiled and nodded. He hadn't said I was too old or fat or that running would ruin my knees. In the past, when asked why I quit running, I'd say "I blew out my knees." In truth, I gave up from exhaustion. What I was doing now—easing into it, using intervals, running slower than I thought a human being could—bore little resemblance to my running days of the past. Ed sensed that.

He'd seen me try so many diet and exercise regimens that he probably had to guard against hoping that jogging might help my weight and depression. He may have thought it was another phase, like that of the mini-trampoline gathering dust in the basement. My mother had given it to us after it had become a clothes rack at her house. I'd bounced on it religiously for six weeks before the activity grew so boring, I gave up.

I took his lack of questions not as a failure of interest, but a silence caused by his reserved nature. No comment was akin to approval. Plus, he knows how even praise can spin my mind, morphing it into pressure. His stoic encouragement gave me the propulsion to continue.

But the morning I was to attempt week three, I woke thinking, "I can't." In this third week, the training plan doubled the time I jogged. I closed my eyes and tried to go back to sleep.

My first few seconds of actual consciousness had been fraught with terrifying projections: me in a black dress at Ed's funeral or a veterinarian plunging the fatal needle into Morgan's forepaw. Next came a litany of unpleasant memories: my niece struggling with crutches after her leg was amputated, my mother begging for water before her final surgery, the grip of my father's hand as a nurse installed a catheter.

In my half-conscious state, I barely noticed Ed opening the bedroom door and leaning down to kiss me goodbye before he left for work. I only half felt Morgan jump onto the bed and curl behind my knees. I snuggled around him, careful not to move too much so he wouldn't jump down.

Five years before, when Mom met Morgan, she'd said, "You'd pay a hairdresser good money for those highlights," referring to the beige and rust "angel wings" pattern on his back. Animal Control had found the one-year-old yellow Lab near a freeway interchange. His good looks, combined with kennel cough and excellent behavior, kept him out of the pound and possibly saved his life. They sent him to a veterinarian who fostered dogs. Enough time had passed since our golden retriever, Bodhi, had died that Ed and I were ready for another canine family member. Ed contacted the vet, who brought Morgan to our house for a test visit. While I feared someone was ugly-crying about losing him, after watching the handsome young dog chase a tennis ball in our fenced backyard for half an hour, Ed called the veterinarian and told her not to bother coming back. Mom believed Morgan had escaped when his owners were traveling. She might have been right. Unlike our previous dogs, Morgan whined and cried in the car. In every other respect, he was the consummate gentleman, even so young. He was housebroken, knew all his commands, only destroyed the occasional sofa pillow, and wove himself seamlessly into our lives and hearts.

The warmth and pressure of Morgan's body pushed away the unpleasant images that had haunted me when I'd first awakened. I peeked out from under the covers at the 1950s mirrored closet doors to see his brown eyes staring back. He stretched out to his full length and thwacked his tail against me, reminding me that some of us are still alive. I am loved and cared for by a good dog, a great man, loving family members, and friends. I rolled over and lifted the covers from my head.

***

I headed to the bathroom. As I sat on the toilet, Mr. Dawg brushed his whiskers against my face. Some people insist that dogs smell your breath from times when wolf mothers returned to the den to throw up a bellyful of food for the puppies to eat. Not my Morgan. He put his snout just close enough to my mouth that I could feel his whiskers graze my lips in the softest gesture. No sloppy kisses or wet jowls from him. His touch was like being tickled for an instant. He may or may not have sniffed, but I doubt he expected me to vomit.

With the snuffling complete, he rubbed against my knees then wiggled beneath my legs against the toilet. Once wedged there, he waited for me to scratch him. He preferred that I scratch between his shoulder blades, as if the identification microchip was working its way out. I worried about these things. My job was to scratch up and down his back with both hands, fingernails digging into his flat, stiff fur. When satisfied, he walked away and curled into a donut shape on the bathroom rug. That was my signal to get off the toilet. Since he had become my trainer and cheerleader, I needed to keep him happy, so I obeyed.

Our "dog therapy" complete, I was ready to face week three. I dressed, picked up the timer, leashed the dog, and went outside.

His comforting presence gave me enough courage to start on our street. I hit the timer. When it was time for double the amount of jogging (three full minutes!), I bent my knees, began slowly, and paced myself. After what I was sure was three minutes, winded, but not exhausted, I checked the timer. Two minutes and thirty seconds. I could do thirty more seconds.

The intervals passed quickly. During the walking periods, I wished I were jogging. During the jogging, I wondered when it would be time to walk again. When we finished, I was sweatier and more tired than the week before. I needed a nap.

We repeated this combination two more times to complete week three.

Each day I grew stronger. I'd needed a nap after day one, but after day two, I thought about a nap, but didn't take one. By day three, napping didn't come to mind. The haranguing in my head continued, but I told the nasty voice, "Listen. You keep telling me I can't, but I AM. Please shut up!" This silenced it for a while, then it returned with more lies. But now, I wasn't believing them.

***

I didn't know running was in our genes. My father, a tall, thin, long-legged German, looked like a marathoner. As the anchor of his high school mile-relay team, he had won the state championship, and set a record that stood for many years. Eventually, my sister gave me his medals.

My uncle on my mother's side also ran, but he's built with short legs and a long body. When we visit, he reminisces about his glory days as a runner. His favorite distance was the 10k (6.2 miles), which he said was, "long enough to get yourself warmed up, but not far enough to kill you."

I was a normal-sized child, despite feeling fat. I only gained considerable weight when, in my thirties, I went on antidepressants. I have my father's long legs and arms, but a short body. If I had my uncle's long torso as well, I would be six feet tall.

***

The trail shoes I'd worn during my first three weeks of training were heavy and hot. I'd need something lighter soon.

Two years before, in 2008, I'd tried to run in sandals. I'd just graduated from MFA school and had gained twenty pounds, eating over that stress combined with the deaths of my niece and mother. In the sandals, my ankle swelled to the size of a grapefruit. An urgent-care doctor said it was my weight. He echoed my self-deprecation. So, once again, I quit. But now, despite my previous swollen-ankle mishap and the fact that I still carried the weight, I thought I wanted "proper" running sandals.

I drove to the same running store I'd gone to years before. My friend then had said, "You need the right equipment." But I'd been a starving law student and had left empty-handed. Today, I entered the store determined to buy the right equipment.

When I asked for running sandals, the young sales clerk screwed up her face. She showed me Vibram five fingers, essentially gloves for your feet. I screwed up my face. "It's for minimalist runners," she said.

I didn't know what a minimalist runner was, so I asked her to suggest something else. I mentioned my previously swollen ankle, but not my weight. I looked nothing like the thin employees or other customers.

"Let me watch you walk without shoes," she said. I walked and felt self-conscious as she studied my gait.

She also measured my foot in the Brannock device they've been measuring feet with since the dawn of time. "Your feet will swell when you run. Go at least a half size larger," she said. Her tone of expertise impressed me, even though she was young enough to be my dead niece.

"Try them out in the parking lot," she suggested. I hadn't worn the sports bra, and, since I could barely tolerate being seen in my own neighborhood, I declined and just walked around the store.

The large, cushioned shoes felt like walking in marshmallow clown boots. "Beginning runners need more support," she said. I'd gone in looking for sandals. These were the opposite. Having done no research, I didn't know the running shoe trend was toward more flexible, lower-heeled shoes as an alternative to the highly cushioned and immobilizing shoes she recommended. I said I'd take them.

Form-fitting tops, stretch tights, and split shorts hung on racks around me. I hadn't researched running clothes either, so I also didn't know that "cotton kills," and turned away from those and toward a wall of ankle socks in different fabrics, thicknesses, and colors. My tube socks had to go. I chose the same brand I'd used to try on the shoes. With pads under the toes and ball of the foot, and on the heel, plus a stretchy, colored material across the top, they added to the pillowy feel. I bought three pairs: aqua to match the shoes, pale pink, and black.

I'd just spent more money on running gear in one hour than I'd spent on any clothing in the last few years. When I was younger and thinner (and possibly hypomanic), I easily dropped hundreds of dollars on work clothes, but weight gain, lack of energy, and practically nonexistent self-worth had driven me out of the stores. Now, I peeked into the bag and smiled at the small bit of color on the socks. I was a serious jogger!

***

A few days later, after jogging, I had coffee with my friend Krista.

As I slid into a booth, she pointed to my workout pants and asked if I'd been exercising. While I was still depressed enough not to shower regularly, another measurement of my mental health, I hadn't sweated enough to warrant the effort.

Krista was a few years older than me and exercised regularly. In the past, when she suggested exercise might improve my emotional well-being, I gave her the responses I used to ward off such recommendations. "I'm tired. It's cold. I'm fat. It will ruin my knees. I don't like exercise. I don't have the energy." I didn't think of these as excuses. I thought myself incapable. There had been a day when I exercised, and that day had passed.

My attitude was changing.

"I'm jealous," she said. She had run races and now walked her Jack Russell terrier and bicycled. Running, she said, hurt her knees.

Every story about how hard running was on the knees made me wonder if there wasn't a better way to run. In the unlikely event that I ran longer distances, I might research it.

"You should do Race for the Cure," Krista suggested.

"Um, no," I said, nearly knocking over my coffee. "I'm not leaving the neighborhood."

She added, "Races are like parties for people who exercise. Plus, you raise money for charity."

"I'm not even sure I'll stick with it," I said, trying to derail her.

"I waddle," I said. I hadn't yet stumbled onto John Bingham's "waddling penguin" society, but that's how I thought I looked.

She did not understand how I'd struggled just to jog where the neighbors might look out their windows. I had friends who dressed in pink clothes and wigs to run or walk 3.1 miles to raise money for breast cancer research with twenty thousand others. I wasn't one of them.

"I'm a private runner," I said, remembering the pleasant intervals in the neighborhood with the dog. I'd begun to think of it as therapy.

Undeterred, Krista told me about her son's training schedule when he'd run the Akron Marathon. He did three or four short runs during the week and a longer run on the weekend. Each week, the long run distance increased, until he was running about twenty miles. Before the race, he "tapered," cutting back his mileage "to rest up."

While it sounded grueling, his marathon training intrigued me. I was following my own training plan. With a plan, I don't have to think. I just follow the schedule. This might be why I like meditation and writing practice so much. You set the timer and sit or write. No second-guessing. Hearing about her son's training plan made my schedule more legitimate.

When I explained that I didn't know how far I was walking and jogging, Krista also told me about a tracking website. Years ago, I used my car's odometer to calculate how far I ran. Now, using Google Maps, the site tells how far you ran. You enter how long it took, and it calculates the pace. This seemed like more information than I needed, but I couldn't wait to go home and try.

CHAPTER 3

Fellowship

My first glimpse of the running community came in "Calling All Penguins (Slow Runners)," a beginner forum thread on the website active.com. Here, I discovered John Bingham, a writer for *Runner's World Magazine*, whose column, "No Need for Speed," and books encouraged runners of all types, despite slowness, awkwardness, or other limiting thoughts. He described thinking that his reflection in a store-front window made him look more like a penguin than the athlete he felt he was. The moniker stuck.

Runners on the thread waddled or "wogged" or "woggled" or plodded. When I posted that I had completed week three, "irunforbling" replied, "Great job! On to week four!" About my shoe and sock purchase, "slowbutsure" said, "Never enough gear!" I felt at home. Even though I didn't want to run with (or in front of) people and told my friend Krista I wouldn't race, it was nice to meet other inexperienced runners without having to leave the house. I needed support.

***

I'd grown up mostly alone. By the time I was born, Mom and Dad were in their thirties. My brother and sister escaped to their adult lives before I finished middle school. My drinking parents fought over money. Occasional outbursts of temper punctuated their brooding silences. To isolate and zone out, I practiced flute in my room, cantered solo around the yard pretending I was a horse, or escaped to the woods to build "cities" from fallen trees. I tried to stay out of the way, but developed a veil of sadness, and extreme negative thinking. In my teen years, I binge-drank.

Alcohol blurred the sharp edges of life, and drinking felt as natural as breathing. My parents allowed me to drink openly with them long before I learned to drive. Our family measured distances and projects by the number of beers they would take. The utility room never contained fewer than three cases of long-necked Budweisers, and the bottom refrigerator drawer (which I would learn in college most families filled with vegetables) we reserved for chilling the beer.

At sixteen, I passed out at a Heart concert on the floor of the women's bathroom and promptly swore off alcohol only to start drinking again a few weeks later. Into college and law school, with each consequence, I would quit, then soon forgot that even the first drink was a bad idea. I lost the car more than once. In a blackout, I slugged a friend. While working at the law firm, I rolled a brand-new station wagon. I wound up in situations and with people I shouldn't have, even though my binges were sometimes years apart.

Finally, one night when I was in my thirties, I stood in front of an open refrigerator negotiating with the six-pack that sat on the middle shelf. I knew where it would end. I sought help, and a community of ex-problem drinkers taught me how to stay stopped. Without those fellow travelers, I was doomed.

***

The Penguins became my running fellowship. When I wrote about conquering the hill near the ravine by our house, they cheered. They talked about shoes, water (hydration) belts, sports bras, tech shirts, capris, and underwear. They talked about interval training, long slow runs, tempo runs—all new to me. *Fartlek*? Is that even a word? They explained that "fartlek" is Swedish for "speed play." You "play" with speed, altering your pace on a whim.

As my knowledge grew, so did my confidence. Soon, I too was posting "WTG!" if a newcomer reported progress. The people in the Penguin Forum couldn't see my middle-aged body as I slogged through my neighborhood. I might be shy in front of other people, but not on the internet. I eagerly shared what I had learned.

With the Penguins, I began to think of myself as a runner. Never mind that I was barely running five minutes at a time. Depression makes me think I'm worthless, that the good days are behind me, and only doom and gloom lie ahead. By taking myself more seriously, I put in more effort and was less likely to quit. I hoped others would take me seriously too, but that wasn't as important as me remembering a competence I thought I lacked. In my slow, middle-aged way, I was good at running. Sharing my limited experience kept the dangerously dull mood at bay, at least while I was on the Penguin Forums.

**

My joy was short-lived. The last week of April, as I completed week four, my ankle swelled the way it had so many years before. When it remained swollen a few days later, it scared me enough to stop.

Over the next two weeks, the dog and I took many long walks, but it broke my heart to think I would lose the fitness and fun. My friends Kim and Fiona continued to post and email about their running. The Penguin Forums just made me sad. I talked to my psychiatrist about a med change, but we held off to see if the darkness would pass.

**

My current psychiatrist and I are vigilant about not letting the darkness linger. We know how bad it can get. In 1994, after I took a disability leave of absence from work, my motivation and joy for life, including the intense running I was doing, faded. Even breathing was difficult.

On a September day, I took the dogs for a run. Weak, worn down, and empty inside, I only managed a block. Running had become a chore, one more thing depression had stolen. I turned the dogs for home. Inside, I took off my running shoes and put them in the back of the closet.

A few days later, stone cold sober, I lay on the family room floor, my heavy head resting on the Berber carpet while Ed was at work. Astro and Maxine, the two dogs I had before Ed and I married, curled around me. My arms, legs, and head felt like they had weights attached, and my mind was thick with sludge. The smallest tasks made me feel as if I were drowning. Outside the family room window, even the blue sky looked bleak.

As I lay there, I imagined loading Maxine, a black Labrador, and Astro, an American Eskimo Dog, into my station wagon, turning on the engine without opening the garage door, and crawling in the back with them. Permanent "sleep" seemed the only reasonable solution. Despite Ed's love, I believed he would be better off without us.

Before I could carry out my fatal plan, the phone rang. I'd forgotten about my psychologist appointment. Still in my pajamas, I went, told her of my plan, and was admitted to the locked ward of a psychiatric hospital until the suicidal thoughts passed. I spent the next six months in various outpatient mental health treatment programs.

With that nervous breakdown, I left the legal profession permanently after ten years of practice. I haven't held a regular job since. I began to write and found homes for a few articles and essays, but low energy and perfectionism kept me from finishing anything longer. I posted occasional articles to my writing blog, *Bum Glue* ("Apply to seat of pants. Sit. Write."), taught a few writing classes, and published a monthly email of Ohio writing events, the *Write Now Newsletter*, working those around my inability to get out of bed and the voices in my head that told me everything I wrote was horrible. I also wrote drafts of three novels, four memoirs, a book about writing, and a book of daily mindfulness meditations. But I couldn't channel the energy to complete those. After several revisions, I decided each book was too flawed and started a new one—nine times. When people asked about work, I said I was retired.

In much the same way that the ex-problem drinkers have kept me on the sober path and various groups of meditators supported my mindfulness practice, the writing community helped me keep pen to page despite my challenges. The Buddhists call their community the "Sangha." Sitting in a quiet room with others provided structure as I attempted to focus on my breath. Discussing the writings of Buddhist teachers brought us together. In writing, critique groups, writing groups (both in person and online), and workshops and conferences allowed me to mingle with other "scribblers." With the recovering people, I learned how to live without alcohol. Beyond mere camaraderie, group synergy made any journey more pleasant, and provided friendly peer pressure and support in tough times. I found these same virtues among the running "Penguins."

***

After two weeks of rest from running, my ankle returned to normal. Perhaps I was ready for week five after all. I mulled that for a few more days before pulling out the schedule. The first day simply increased the amount of jogging and decreased the walk breaks. But the second day required eight minutes of jogging, and the third day jumped to a steady twenty minutes straight with, get this, no walking! I panicked. If I couldn't do the second or third day, why bother with the first?

No, this thinking does not make sense, but that's how my mind works. For fifteen minutes, I tried to convince myself to just do the first day. I tried to recall the increased energy and happy mood the workouts produced. I tried to imagine myself succeeding, but the panic would not subside. I'd expected each week to follow the same format, with an increased challenge to be repeated three times. I sulked, unable to make myself put on exercise clothes, leash up the dog, or do anything productive. Blue and mildly nauseous, I called a friend, but she didn't answer. I called Ed, but he was busy with work. I surfed the internet and played many games of computer solitaire. The day passed, and I did not even try.

***

The next day, I reluctantly dragged myself out of bed. I trust someone's experience more than their opinion, so I logged into the Penguin Forum to ask about week five. "It's a big shift," one person who had also found it daunting said. She encouraged me to just try day one and see how it went.

Two weeks had passed since I'd completed the week four workouts. My ankle had swollen. I'd concluded jogging wasn't for me.

Her suggestion reminded me of how much better I'd felt after the previous workouts—almost like an athlete. Maybe I should attempt it. When I remembered I was supposed to be talking myself out of it, I laughed.

The dog found no humor in it. If I walked near the table on which sat the little timer, his ears perked up. When I didn't touch it, his ears fell and my heart broke. Maybe, with Mr. Dawg by my side, I'd succeed.

Down in the ravine, two run/walk intervals left me gasping for air. There would be no third. I turned the dog for home once again. At the house, I crawled into bed. The dog hopped up and curled behind my knees.

Before I fell asleep, I remembered that a Penguin had said he'd repeated a few of the weeks. At the time when I'd read his comment, I hadn't been able to start week five at all. The thought of repeating week five wasn't helpful.

But wait. I could repeat week four! This wasn't a sprint. It was its own marathon. I didn't want to give up, the way I had in my previous attempts to run. I wanted to be a lifetime runner. If I ever chose to race, maybe I'd win my age group when I was in my nineties by being the only one to take part. Of course, I never intended to race, but...

The following day, I began again. Over the next three weeks, I repeated the week four intervals three times a week until the set was easy. Maybe week five would happen after all.

***

Once the week four workouts felt comfortable, I turned back to the three different workouts of week five. The third workout culminated in twenty minutes of continuous jogging. TWENTY MINUTES! I'd told the Penguins I was in for the long haul, but still felt confused at how to continue.

Morgan lay on the floor next to my desk joyfully ripping a scarlet and gray rope toy into pieces.

Pieces! That was it.

I'd break week five into three pieces ("week 5A," "week 5B," and "week 5C"), then repeat each one until it was easy. I hugged Morgan's stiff fur, inhaling his doggy smell.

With Morgan smiling beside me, I set out to complete day one of week 5A. I huffed and puffed. This was difficult AND I was doing it.

When it was time for the final five-minute jog, I was back to the steep hill at the edge of the ravine. Burning bush glowed with the fresh green of spring. Dogwoods and redbuds would soon bloom. The world would be beautiful if I made it up this hill.

Even at a slow jog, my breath came in rasps. The dog pulled and the distance between us tugged at my heart. I slowed, caught my breath, and began to jog again, closing the distance between the dog and me. Never mind that he was walking; I wasn't going to let him beat me to the top. I dug deep, and we crested the hill together. I looked at the timer. Three minutes still to go.

"Walking is not a failure," I told the dog, and let my heart rate slow. The rest of the street was still uphill, but more gradual. At the stop sign, I resumed jogging. "We can do this," I told Morgan. He nodded, or maybe shook a bug off his ear. Panting again, I slowed to what must have looked like a crawl to the people not watching from their houses. I passed one house, then another, turned a corner and passed more. Stucco house. Siding house. Brick house. Maple tree. Crabapple. Dogwood. Tiny buds would soon flower. One more minute. Eight more seconds. Then the sweet beep.

Day one of week 5A, done. "Whoop! Whoop!" I yelled, startling the dog. I patted him and gave myself a mental pat, too.

***

As a new runner, I'd been blissfully unaware that some faster runners resent slower people. But one night, as I scrolled through the Penguin Forums, I read, "You slow runners are pathetic. If I ran as slow as you did, I'd shoot myself." The condescension turned my stomach. "I reported you to the moderators," I replied.

The troll responded by using my account photo to clone my account by adding one letter to the end of my name. I'd naively used my real name, and a photo of me with Mr. Dawg as my avatar. The troll wrote critical posts about other members of the forum under this new account which, at a brief glance, looked like mine. He also looked up my Twitter account and website and criticized those. The forum moderators took down the troll's comments and account, but the troll continued. From then on, I didn't engage, but simply clicked the "report abuse" button. I also changed my username, password, and photo. But I didn't leave.

The troll claimed that anyone not placing in their age groups shouldn't race. He complained of having to dodge slow runners who mistakenly started too far in front. I hadn't raced, so I didn't know the norms, but these comments made me even more reluctant. Some Penguins talked about being asked to move to the sidewalk, being picked up in a vehicle because they were too slow, or finishing last. I doubled down on my intent to only run in private, with the dog, through the streets of our neighborhood.

***

Toward the end of July, in an email exchange, I finally told my sister about running. I qualified it with the fact that I was interspersing walking and hadn't yet run an entire thirty minutes.

Since 2007, the year her daughter, our mother, my father-in-law, and her ex-husband died, Amy and I have texted each other every day. Like my husband, she has seen me through the trials of mental illness. I've seen her through divorce, her own depression, and the death of her only child. We cling to each other like survivors of an emotional shipwreck. Time passed, and I forgot I'd told her. She walks her dog and swims, but never expressed interest in sports beyond the Ohio State University Buckeyes.

Just when I had recommitted to never running in public, she emailed a link to the first annual Steps for Sarcoma 5k. It would raise money for research to combat osteosarcoma, the type of cancer that had killed my niece. Amy was walking the one-mile fun walk.

"Would you run the 5k?" she asked.

"Oh, no," I wrote. "Running is a private thing."

I didn't think of this as a cop-out. I really didn't think I could bear being seen running in public. Plus, my ankle still swelled intermittently.

But each time I went out to jog, thoughts of my niece's death nearly suffocated me.

Jamey had been a runner. Until she was diagnosed with a cancerous tumor in her femur, she thought the pain in her leg was a running injury. If she were still alive, she would be running. Even after her leg was amputated, she tried to wear a prosthetic limb, hoping to run again.

I had told my sister I wouldn't participate, but held it in the back of my mind.

My training and the Penguins forum buoyed my confidence. When my sister asked again, I reconsidered.

The Penguins posted race finish times in the signatures to their posts. I had not yet timed myself, so didn't know my pace. I was afraid to know. But I kept reading about them collecting race bibs and crossing the finish line even if it was last. The trolls popped in from time to time, but as quickly disappeared. One race might not hurt.

Meanwhile, I asked my friend Krista more about races. She teased me for saying I'd never do one. The idea of supporting a cause I found important changed my perspective. She also found races fun. Raising money for a cause gave her a sense of purpose. She said I wouldn't finish last and, even if I did, I would survive. I don't know why I was so afraid of coming in last, but I was.

Then one day I noticed a 26.2 sticker on the back of a friend's car. Now that I was running, even at my snail's pace, these white, oval stickers appeared on my radar. To me, the 26.2 sticker was the equivalent of a Ph.D. diploma for running. I already had three college degrees (bachelor's, master's, and Juris Doctor) and several academic and license certificates. I wanted to add this achievement to my collection. My friend's was the first 26.2 sticker I'd noticed on the car of someone I knew.

I caught my young friend and asked about his running. Tall and lean, he looked the way I thought a marathoner should. Standing outside the building where we both attended a recovery group, I confided, "I'd like to earn my own 26.2 sticker someday." I looked at the ground, waiting for the, "You've got to be kidding" look. Instead, he smiled. "Keep running, and in time you'll do it." My throat closed. I was easily twice his age, much heavier, and hadn't even run a 5k. I was probably manic. No matter. This kind man believed in me.

I didn't tell my sister, but planned for the 5k.

CHAPTER 4

A Perfect Storm

Weight loss and the looming prospect of the "Big Five-Oh!" would have been enough reason for me to take up running again. There was also that wacky recurring dream. But these were surface factors. In fact, the seeds of Kim and Fiona's posts landed on ground made fertile by difficulties starting five years before. A perfect storm of life events had created the critical mass necessary to get me off the sofa.

Still, I wanted to lose weight.

In high school and my twenties, I might gain five pounds during the winter, but easily lost that in the spring. By my early thirties, I looked anorexic. For the six months before I met Ed, I coped with the stress of practicing law with stringent diets. Chunks of my hair fell out, and I was frequently lightheaded, while my period stopped completely. The first time Ed opened the refrigerator in my house, it contained only an expired bottle of ketchup, a bag of apples, and a sleeve of bagels. By that time, I was only eating one bagel and one apple, cut into thirds, each day.

After my nervous breakdown, I could no longer summon the effort required to control my food. When I began taking antidepressants, the obsession transformed into overeating and yo-yo dieting, which packed on the weight. By my early forties, the scale hit two hundred pounds. I joined a recovery group for food issues and lost nearly forty pounds, but when I saw Kim's posts about running, I was far from happy with my size.

I'd gone off antidepressants several times to lose weight. The weight came off, but the depression, anxiety, and panic attacks came back so viciously that, within a few months, I was back at the psychiatrist's, begging for a prescription. My most recent experiment with quitting meds, just a year before I took up running, had also failed. I went back on the drugs, but it takes several months for my antidepressant to take effect, so once again, I missed nine months of well-being for the sake of twenty pounds.

I knew from my previous exercise stints that depression hates a moving target. I'd taken Nia dance classes in 2004 and 2005. I would ease in, but before class ended, I was jumping, kicking, and panting like a fiend. Happy at accomplishing something, I left the class hypomanic, which felt like an improvement.

But when our golden retriever Bodhi died, I couldn't bring myself to dance. I took long, slow, dogless walks, mourning my canine friend, or escaped the silent house to write in coffee shops. The solace of summer air, wind in the trees, and the swing of my arms was the best medicine. Happily, when Morgan joined our family, he became my walking companion and canine therapist.

***

On a September day, just a month after we adopted Mr. Dawg, Mom called to say Jamey was being admitted to Children's Hospital.

At the hospital, my twenty-one-year-old niece lay on the bed in a "spica" cast that covered all of one leg and half her body up to her waist. The room purred with the hushed voices of her friends. They were students at Ohio State University, coworkers, and high school classmates. More than a dozen of them filled all the chairs, every inch of floor space, and the windowsill. My sister and the rest of our family sat in stunned silence in a meeting room across the hall.

The young people took turns signing her cast. When a young man offered me a package of markers, Jamey brushed a blonde hair away from her eyes and said, "Write something, Aunt Nita." I pulled out the purple one and, just beneath where her toes peeked out, scrawled, "Here. Now."

The pain meds hadn't knocked her out the way the medical staff thought they should. Her tolerance would also prove too high to dull the pain to come.

I pointed at her toes and said, "When you get scared, remember there's only this moment and I'm with you." I felt so helpless and pathetic trying to apply mindfulness techniques to her situation, but she smiled.

When Mom had called, I'd asked, "Why Children's? She's twenty-one."

The cancer she had, osteosarcoma, usually strikes teens. The doctors at Children's were the experts. The tumor in Jamey's thigh had likely been growing for months. By the time an MRI found it that morning, it had broken her femur, the largest and strongest bone in the body. Ultimately, that tumor and the lesions already in her lungs would also break our hearts.

Jamey had been five when her parents divorced, and, because funds were short, I'd taken her shopping. We'd walked the aisles of the big-box store hand in hand, choosing first a frilly, pink, impractical dress that made her eyes shine. Then we filled the cart with underwear, socks, T-shirts, pants, shoes, and a warm coat, all the things she needed to start school. This shopping trip and the few birthday parties I attended had been the best I could do. I spent the precious time I now wished I had devoted to her, and the rest of my family, drafting legal documents and priding myself on the number of hours I billed. I had never wanted children of my own, but thought of her as the next best thing to a daughter. I vowed to be there when she or Amy needed me.

***

In 2006, while Jamey was sick, I enrolled in Goddard College's non-residential Master of Fine Arts (MFA) program in Creative Writing. I chose Goddard because they could accommodate my mental health issues. Between residencies, and when I wasn't at Jamey's, I lived at my desk or on the sofa reading and writing. I drank large decaf soy lattes every day. While completing the assignments gave me a sense of accomplishment, I gained weight and lost touch with the positive body sensations exercise had brought.

During the July 2006 residency, Amy called. I had to excuse myself from the classroom at Fort Worden to go outside to get phone reception. As I stood on the grassy lawn, I listened as my sister wept into her phone back in Ohio. "It's in her spine!" she shrieked. I sank to the grassy lawn and sobbed, unable to maintain the composure I wished I could keep to calm my sister.

By November, the tumor in Jamey's leg had stopped the circulation to her foot. She had to have her leg amputated. After the surgery, she called from the ICU in agony. Because of her high tolerance for medications, normal doses weren't blocking the excruciating pain. "Tell me how to meditate," she begged. I guided her through a basic body scan. As I talked, possibly from the drugs finally working, she went to sleep. My sister took the phone and thanked me.

In February 2007, Jamey died. She was twenty-four. Her death turned the natural order of the world on its ear and plummeted me into despair. I began having panic attacks again and took to my bed.

***

For the rest of 2007, grief blasted Ed and me as if from a fire hose.

In July, one of Ed's good friends and former coworkers died.

In August, Ed's ninety-six-year-old father died.

In September, the man my mother had dated after my father's death died.

In October, both Jamey's cat and Jamey's father died.

In November, Mom's best friend died.

With each death, I thought, "This is it for a while." I imagined burning my black dress.

But 2007 wasn't finished with us yet.

***

In 1996, when he was sixty-seven, my father died of metastatic lung cancer. After his doctor told him to "get his affairs in order," I spent as much time with him as I could, golfing, traveling, and sitting by his bedside when he and my mother moved in with me and Ed during

Dad's final months. I grieved his death, but that loss did little to prepare me for 2007.

I was at a writing retreat with Natalie Goldberg in New Mexico when Amy called to say our seventy-seven-year-old mother had been admitted to a central Ohio hospital with a bowel obstruction. "But she was just dog-sitting Morgan!" I protested. She had seemed fine when I left town.

Illness plagued Mom her entire life. She spent hours in bed, behind the closed bedroom door. I would pull a wooden chair up to the kitchen counter near the toaster and put in the bread. When I had buttered the toast perfectly, the way Dad taught me, I would take it to her in exchange for a smile. Many of her illnesses were real, but others remained a mystery, as doctor after doctor couldn't find the cause of her symptoms. I grew up worried she was on the verge of death.

And her mood swings were legend. Undiagnosed bipolar disorder aggravated by drinking compounded her hypochondria. She alternated between clinging possessiveness and near-abandonment. I never knew which mother to expect. When I came home from school, she might be pounding out tunes on the organ at a volume that rattled the windows, aiming to throw a potholder at me, or in bed, paralyzed by negative thoughts and alcohol. She stopped drinking after I was an adult, and we healed many of our wounds, but I still found her confusing and unpredictable.

After Dad died, I spent countless hours with her in medical waiting rooms as they treated her for diabetes, C.O.P.D., and a chronic cough. I lived closest and didn't have a day job. Despite my protests that I wasn't her "primary caretaker," when she asked, I packed my laptop and headphones and did my best to write in the lobby. Every crisis seemed fatal, but each time she survived. She'd even been hospitalized for a bowel obstruction before, but it resolved without surgery. When Amy called, part of me rolled my eyes wondering if this was another imaginary illness. Regardless, I got on the next plane.

When the obstruction hadn't cleared after five days, they took her to surgery. Ed, Amy, Jim, Deanna, and I sat in the gray hospital waiting room. I tried to read but couldn't. We talked about things I can't remember. I ate a lot of snacks. After many hours, the surgeon greeted us, smiling. Adhesions had strangled her small intestine and shut off blood flow to one area. He had freed her intestines from the tangle of scar tissue and that section had "pinked back up." Confident it would heal, he decided against resecting it. "He's the doctor" I told myself. I would not want to second-guess him.

The days in the hospital wore on and on. Still in graduate school, I wrote annotations by her bedside. Day after day, she remained in her bed, while other patients who'd had the same surgery were up and walking the halls. When the doctors or nurses visited, we advocated for her, but frankly, the deaths that year had worn me down.

One night, when I came home from another long day at the hospital, Ed asked me to come into his office. He pointed to his computer. On the screen was an article about adhesions. "Her prognosis isn't good," he said. I shook my head, cried "She will be fine!" then stomped off to bed, sobbing.

After she had been in the hospital twenty-four days, her intestines remained blocked and became infected. The doctor called for a second surgery. As her medical power of attorney, I again signed the forms warning about the dangers of surgery. As a lawyer, I'd seen many releases, but my hands shook as I signed this one.

Before the hospital staff wheeled her back, Amy, Jim, Deanna, and I stood around her bed. Her tiny frame, now thin from so many days on a liquid diet, lay in a mass of tangled sheets. With speech slurred from pain and anxiety medications, she called out, "I know you all think I'm a pain!" We laughed and groaned, "Oh, Mom!" She was right, but we still loved her. I remembered how she had encouraged me to learn to play the flute despite my anxiety. I could see her at the kitchen table, cutting fabric I'd chosen for a top. I could hear her singing "Happy Birthday" in her sweet soprano. I couldn't let her go into surgery thinking we hated her. I went to her side. "You gave me my creativity," I said. "Thank you." I kissed her and they took her away.

Back in that gray waiting room, we sat again, hour after hour. When the doctor finally came out, I stood. Nervous, I made an awkward joke about how much faster this surgery had been. He glared, his face a stone.

"She's not going to survive this," he said.

My knees buckled and I stumbled backward into the gray chair where moments before I'd had hope. Deanna gripped my arm. I covered my face with my hands and tried to listen, but the doctor's words spun through my mind on repeat:

She's not going to survive this.

She's not going to survive this.

She's not going to survive.

He had not expected to find Mom's small intestine disintegrated. "It was like wet tissue paper," he said. Nothing to salvage. Jim, Amy, Deanna, and Ed all asked questions as I stared at the gray wall. Surely the doctor was wrong.

As it turns out, you can't live without your small intestine. If it's not there to absorb the nutrients, you starve of malnutrition. None of us had any medical training. None of us knew that.

The surgeon's face softened as he asked, "What do you want me to do?" If they treated her infection, she would remain alive, but die of malnutrition in weeks. If they let it go, the fever would kill her more quickly.

Regardless of the questions everyone asked, we knew the only humane answer. Mom, still heavily sedated, was transferred to the hospice wing. The next afternoon, December 30, 2007, we surrounded her while she died peacefully.

As irrational as even I knew it was, I felt responsible for "letting" her die. I hadn't made the toast properly. I hadn't gone to medical school. I hadn't seen it coming. This insane belief, combined with all the previous deaths and the notion that I was now "next in line" for the mortuary, sent me into a spiral. I ate, slept, and cried.

***

I remained stuck for nearly a year after Mom's death and almost two years after we'd lost Jamey. Finally, in November 2008, Morgan and I began to take slow walks around the block. Throughout my years of mood disorders, my long-time friend Lora had used vigorous exercise to treat the depression from her fibromyalgia. Another friend, Pat, had taken up tennis to treat her depression. "You need to break a sweat," they each said. I was skeptical. I'd tried and abandoned so many forms of movement. Plus, when fatigued, the last thing I wanted to do was sweat. I thought about Nia dance classes, but the instructor I loved had stopped teaching, and I didn't have the energy to drive somewhere. I needed something at home. Those long, slow dog walks in the fresh air, along with therapy and recovery groups, started to bring me back to life. When I saw Kim and Fiona's posts, I secretly hoped running would speed the healing.

CHAPTER 5

Wonky Ankle

Shortly after I met Ed, he asked if I wanted to learn to meditate. He'd learned at ten-day Zen retreats before we met. He also did Tai Chi.

Ed set the microwave timer for five minutes. We sat on the stiff dining room chairs I rarely used, and I did my best to focus on my breath.

"My mind races," I said, fidgeting.

"Sit still and focus. It will slow down on its own."

Over the next two decades, I built up to long periods of sitting, in much the same way as I was now acclimating to running. I'd been a regular meditator for nearly twenty years and experienced much of the calm and concentration Ed had promised.

After I began running, a colleague told me about ChiRunning. The word "chi" means "life force." ChiRunning founder Danny Dreyer used Tai Chi principles to create the technique "to reduce injury and improve personal performance...to help you love running forever." The Eastern philosophy interwoven in the technique aligned with my practice.

I mostly hoped ChiRunning would prevent my ankle from swelling, so I set aside my fear of being seen and took a ChiRunning class with instructor Doug Dapo and two other women students. We spent four hours in a Westerville park, more time than I'd spent outside in years. I learned the hazards of over-striding, the benefits of midfoot landing, and the advantages of "minimalist shoes." The highly cushioned shoes I'd bought might contribute to my ankle problems. I also learned to use a metronome to increase my foot turnover. I went home and ordered the DVD, a metronome, and an audio recording to hear Danny's instructions as I ran.

Doug videotaped us before and after and played back the recordings to compare. I'd known my exercise bra was old, and looser since I'd lost weight, but until I watched a video showing my flopping breasts, I hadn't fully appreciated a good sports bra.

I asked the women Penguins and my running friends for recommendations and researched online. At the store, I tried the brand most recommended, but it had so many hooks and eyes in front that I lost track when I tried to count. I wanted to love it but couldn't get it on. I bought a different one with adjustable straps. It allowed me to breathe but held things in place.

I immediately implemented Doug's suggestion that each run have a "form focus." I often chose "pelvic tilt" because I needed so much improvement in that area. Having a "focus" reminded me of the "object of meditation" one chooses in sitting practice. Each time I ran, if my mind wandered, I brought it back to whatever focus I had chosen for that run, the same way I did while meditating.

***

As I completed weeks five and six of the interval training, my left ankle, the same ankle that swelled in 2008 when I'd tried to run in sandals, grew stiff and swollen around the bone. Back then, I'd attributed it to weight and bad shoes. I now had good shoes and was ten pounds lighter. I shouldn't be jogging at all.

This left ankle never bent the way the right one did. It was larger, and my left toes often cramped. I rested two days and the swelling subsided. But after the next workout, it swelled again. I massaged, iced, and elevated. A normal person might have called a doctor, but I come from a long line of folks who distrust traditional medicine.

In July, on a trip to San Antonio for a convention, Ed and I walked the downtown and River Walk. My ankle had swollen on the plane. The next morning, it was still swollen. I went to the gym to walk on the treadmill. Despite my usual aversion to them, I climbed aboard one and lost myself in the expansive view of the city from the windows. Sturdy and quiet, the treadmill whirred as I ran much further and faster than the training plan said. I climbed off, dizzy and in pain.

My ankle throbbed. When we flew on to Cancun a few days later, it swelled more. A massage and a wrap at the spa reduced the swelling, but it didn't go down completely until, back home, I'd rested for a few days. I took an entire week off to ice and elevate it. Again, I worried my jogging days were over.

With the swelling gone, I restarted the training plan at week two, alternating ninety seconds of running with two minutes of walking for twenty minutes. The next day, manic, I ran thirty minutes straight. My ankle ballooned.

***

During July and into early August, when my ankle continued to swell, I called the doctor. Sitting on her examining table, I proclaimed how much I loved "running." The Penguins suggested I call it that instead of "jogging."

I hoped my enthusiasm would spill over to my doctor, but she frowned at my swollen ankle. It wasn't that swollen, the size of a tennis ball instead of a softball. But it was tender near the ankle bone. I worried I'd go home in the boot of shame.

I asked the doctor about gout. People from the farmlands of rural Ohio, where I grew up, blamed gout when their ankles swelled. Maybe a dietary change would ward off the swelling. Gout seemed preferable to an injury, but the doctor shook her head and ordered blood tests. It took the nurse three stabs.

The doctor returned and said she would test for autoimmune issues. An alarm went off in my head.

"Autoimmune issues?" I asked, feeling even more lightheaded than I had when the nurse was drawing blood.

"Yes, RA."

"Like arthritis?"

"Yes. You haven't fallen, tripped, or done anything else to sprain it."

I had not.

A woman I knew in college had rheumatoid arthritis. I remembered her swollen joints, low energy level, and pain. Tears stung my eyes.

"It might explain your tiredness and depression too."

No one else had tested me for RA. Maybe there were treatments. Maybe she was wrong. I left the office with an upset stomach and a still-swollen ankle.

***

After that visit to my primary care physician, I modified the training plan to my ability and continued running intervals: run for ten, walk for one, run for ten again. I still hadn't signed up for the 5k.

When my ankle swelled, I assumed I would never run again and grew despondent. After a few days of rest, gentle massage, icing and elevating, the swelling went down and hope returned. Then I would run again. This was the cycle. Run. Swell. Sulk. Ice. Walk. Run. Swell. Sulk. Ice. Walk. Mood swings were my norm, but now they were tied to exercise.

I doubted running would permanently heal my depression, but I craved the runner's rush. In the hours following a run, my arms and legs tingled. My chest and throat opened. The dark heaviness lifted, and my body felt light and warm like an afterglow.

According to a study in the *British Journal of Sports Medicine*, running triggers endocannabinoids, the neurotransmitters stimulated by marijuana. A later study in *Proceedings of the National Academy of Sciences* confirmed this. With runner's high, the world is fine. Everybody loves me. I understand everything. My heart is full. Sound like any drugs you've ever taken? Exactly! That's how I felt, even if I only ran a mile.

I didn't know this science then. Only later would I discover additional science to explain why I was happy when I did my workout and sad when I didn't. My tricky mind continued to tell me I would fail. Each time I achieved a goal, I reminded it that, once again, it didn't know what it was talking about. I began to keep an online running journal and felt another rush when I wrote it down.

Meanwhile, my sister continued to ask me about the 5k.

The next time Mr. Dawg and I ran, when I asked him about the 5k, he perked his copper-colored ears. It's possible he mistook the word "race" for "treat," but I took it as another sign. So what if I came in last? So what if people laughed? So what!

I went home to sign up, but found the website difficult to navigate. Now that I'd changed my mind about racing and the dog had given his approval, the Universe wasn't letting me. Apparently, the dog had been wrong.

I went into the bedroom Ed uses as an office and told him I couldn't sign up. He hugged me and said, "You'll figure it out." After twenty years of my mental trials, he'd learned not to fix me. He asked if I'd emailed the race director. I had.

The next day, the race director and I exchanged more emails. Hours passed. When I finally received a confirmation email, I wrapped my arms around Mr. Dawg and thanked Jamey.

***

In August, I graduated from my trusty kitchen timer to a Timex sports watch. At the running store, a young man showed me the options. There were also GPS watches that track pace, route, and heart rate. I didn't think I needed that much information. He asked about my running and I was embarrassed because of my short mileage, assuming everyone there ran marathons. But he said it was great that I ran at all. I left the store with the watch and another pair of socks because, well, I love socks. And I felt fabulous, like an athlete.

I timed my runs and included the data online, after changing the training schedule to make the intervals easier to track. I'd had a similar watch years before but had killed it in salt water. I'd not replaced it because I wasn't an athlete anymore, and only athletes wore watches like that. Replacing the sports watch was another step in claiming myself as a runner. I vote with my feet by running, but also by where I spend money. I had now spent more on running in a few months than I'd spent on nearly anything in several years.

I ran with the watch for a few weeks before complaining on social media that waiting for Mr. Dawg to pee and poop made my times slower. My friend Wendy, a writer and ultrarunner from Colorado, posted that I could start and stop the watch with the push of a button. Amazing!

***

When Ed told a woman in our book club I was running, she suggested *Born to Run*. "I never thought I'd like a book about running." She said it read like a novel.

I checked the audiobook out of the library and listened in my car. This nonfiction mystery, thriller, and running encyclopedia rolled into one so enthralled me that I'd sit in the garage (with the car off) to listen to the end of a section. It wasn't lost on me that, decades before, I'd sat in a different car in a different garage, trying to summon the courage to kill myself. While those thoughts sometimes still floated through my mind, they no longer threatened to become reality.

In the book, author Chris McDougall sets out on a quest to find ultrarunner Caballo Blanco and the Tarahumara tribe of Mexican Indians, interspersing facts about evolution and the human body. As *ChiRunning* claimed, McDougall found heel-striking and over-striding harmful. McDougall also touted the benefits of chia seeds and eating salad for breakfast. Most important, he claimed human beings are genetically engineered to run.

I was most influenced by Caballo Blanco's instruction to McDougall:

> Think Easy, Light, Smooth, and Fast. You start with easy, because if that's all you get, that's not so bad. Then work on light. Make it effortless, like you don't give a shit how high the hill is or how far you've got to go. When you've practiced that so long that you forget you're practicing, you work on making it smooooooth. You won't have to worry about the last one—you get those three, and you'll be fast.

The book fueled my determination to not let my ankle keep me from running. I'd already experienced what Christopher McDougall described and wanted more. I wanted to run longer distances faster. It helped me mentally prepare for the upcoming 5k.

***

From *Born to Run*, I also learned the history of the running shoe industry. Maybe the shoe industry didn't change models each year to get people to buy multiple pairs in fear of their favorite going out of style, but that was the result. They designed those cushioned, high-heeled running shoes to compensate for heel-striking. Perhaps changing my form and running in minimal shoes would cure my wonky ankle.

The Penguins suggested water shoes, the slip-ons made for water aerobics. Cheaper than trendy minimalist shoes, they were as minimal as you could get without going barefoot. I began to run in those one day a week and walk in them other days, but they quickly wore out. At the sporting goods store, where I went for a sturdier pair, the clerk gaped when I told him I intended to run in them. I explained about the Tarahumara Indians and the research to support minimalist shoes. He shook his head but sold them to me anyway.

***

In the ChiRunning class, Doug explained foot turnover. The average runner's foot turnover is around 150 footfalls per minute. An elite runner's is closer to 180. When a woman asked if that was why elite runners were so much faster, he said yes, but "not for the reason you might think." He showed how his foot turnover stayed the same no matter his pace. "Elites are more efficient." Having your foot on the ground for a shorter period of time uses less energy and is less jarring.

Doug suggested using a metronome to determine our current foot turnover rate and pointed to the small model clipped to his waistband. We were to turn the metronome one beat higher than our current rate and run at that for a week. Once that felt comfortable, we would turn the metronome a beat higher. Gradually increasing the footfalls per minute would not shock our systems, training us to run at a faster cadence with minimal stress. "Gradual progress" is one of the main principles of ChiRunning.

If there's anything I love, it's a good gadget. Like the kitchen timer, the metronome was familiar and friendly. I'd used a much larger one in high school when I played flute. "Beep. Beep. Beep," went the clip-on model, keeping time with Doug's footfalls.

I ordered a gray metronome, less intimidating than black. If they'd had a rhinestone "Hello Kitty" one, I'd have bought that.

Once it came, I clipped it to my waist and leashed up the dog. Again, that old fear of what people thought surfaced, so Mr. Dawg and I jogged to the ravine, where I hoped no one would hear me beeping. Ridiculous, but I didn't entirely believe no one was watching.

In the ravine, the dog tugged when I stopped, but I had to read the instructions. He found a shrub to pee on and a tantalizing scent in the mud. After staring at the contraption, I figured out the volume, mode, and speed. I jogged with my finger on the speed button, and the dog followed. As I jogged, I pushed the button to sync with my footfalls. The number was 153, the cadence of an average jogger.

Doug had used a three-beat rhythm like a waltz: left, two, three, right, two, three, left, two, three. Setting it to beat on each footfall was too fast, but using every other step sometimes resulted in hitting too hard repeatedly on the same foot. I divided my number of footfalls, 153, by three, which equaled fifty-one. In keeping with Doug's gradual progress admonition, I set it for fifty-two, and jogged down the road. Since "more" is always better, part of me wanted to jump to fifty-three. But I remembered "gradual progress." We would take it slow. It was almost time for the 5k.

CHAPTER 6

Running in Public

"I'm looking for packet pickup," I told the running-store clerk. It was the day before my first race, the inaugural Steps for Sarcoma 5k.

A trim young woman smiled knowingly from behind a folding table stacked with T-shirts and plastic bags. She looked up my name, then handed me a T-shirt, a "bib" with my race number, and a plastic sack filled with flyers and four safety pins. I thought I should buy something, but none of their socks appealed, so I left, clutching the bag like a child holding Halloween candy.

To quell my fears, I'd researched race etiquette and asked the Penguins. The safety pins were for the bib. It went on the front. Putting it on the back meant you were an amateur. I was an amateur but wanted no one to know.

Ed and I had driven the course the week before after I'd looked at the race website which had an impressive online course map. I'd only just started using the technology. As we drove the streets of the neighborhood near the park, I imagined myself running them. We walked through the park to get a feel for it.

I'd already walked or run nearly that far. On race day, the bib would be the difference. In addition to my number, 18, the bib bore a computer chip to track when I crossed both the start and finish lines and record my time and pace. Plus, people would be watching. I was still apprehensive about running in public, but willing to try, since it was for a good cause. Ed agreed to take pictures.

The night before the race, I went with friends to an Amish restaurant, where I filled my plate with mashed potatoes and gravy, carb-loading despite the articles I'd read condemning this time-honored tradition.

The articles had been about marathons, not 5ks, but I ate as if it were a marathon.

***

On race morning, a bright autumn day, I made the mistake of saying the word "run" while dressing, and Morgan dashed over. With the dog underfoot, I pulled on my new running bra and a Kelly-green tank which read, "If found on ground, please drag across finish line." I hoped I wasn't borrowing trouble. I pulled on the running shoes, since I didn't think my water shoes were sturdy enough. Plus, someone might think them odd.

We don't call Morgan the "ever-hopeful dog" for nothing. He continued to track me, even as I explained that a race was different. "There might not be other dogs," I said. He parked himself next to the door of "his" closet, where his leash hangs, and gave me his most pathetic look. He only budged when I dropped a few bites of food into his dish to bribe him into the kitchen, where we keep him while we're gone so he doesn't eat the sofa pillows. He gobbled the food. I patted his big, square head and climbed into the car with Ed.

As Ed pulled up to the park, I saw runners with dogs. "I could have brought Morgan," I muttered, but just as quickly said, "Not today." Ed agreed. Better to run this first one solo.

***

My anxiety turned to excitement when I saw the race flags, people milling about, and the inflatable arch marking the start and finish. We gathered near the start with my sister, sister-in-law, surviving niece, her in-laws, and my friends Debbie and Krista. This was the same Krista who I'd told I was a "private runner." My brother would have joined us, but he was out of the country on business.

The little girl inside me imagined the crowd had come to see my first race. This was my graduation from training, completing the journey the dog and I had begun six months before, when I'd run for sixty seconds carrying a digital timer through the ravine. The training takes most people nine weeks. With my wonky ankle and depressed mind, it took me nearly twenty.

But the sadness on my sister's face reminded me why we were there. We would remember those we'd lost, celebrate the survivors, raise money, all while getting exercise. It had been a mere three years since Amy's vibrant daughter was among the living, and the race wouldn't bring Jamey back. My sister and I shared a tearful hug.

***

The Penguins suggested I line up according to pace, in front of the walkers, but behind faster runners. I asked folks their pace. A woman with a baby stroller said, "I'm walking." A man behind her said, "I'm injured, so I'll be slow." I tucked myself between them, and my friends and family joined me. Ed walked past the first turn to wait.

The siren went off, and our chatty group walked across the start line. When we came to where Ed stood, he took a picture then asked, "Aren't you supposed to be running?" I'd forgotten. "I'll see you at the finish!" I sped ahead, but runners weaved around me as I jogged. What kind of runner forgot to run? I shook that off. "Go easy. Just finish."

The course circled the park. Slogans written in chalk on the path cheered, "Beat cancer!" and "Every footstep counts!" People passed. A young girl. Two boys. A woman with a stroller. A woman with a dog. I let them go.

On a small hill, I slowed to thank the police officer who motioned us into a residential neighborhood of two-story houses with manicured lawns. Near the crossing, a cyclist flew toward us, yelling, "Front runners coming through!" The first male, a wiry young man in a singlet and split shorts, sped past the officer and onto the path having already finished the two miles I had yet to go. I didn't know if it was appropriate, but when he passed, I whooped and hollered.

A group of giggling girls in matching "Sarcoma" T-shirts passed me near mile one. My mood sagged. I tried to remember to relax and lean the way Doug, my ChiRunning instructor, had told us, but the street was wide and nearly empty. A handful of walkers followed, but no other runners. I'll be last, I thought, struggling to lift my heavy legs. Then I remembered my goal: have fun and finish upright. On to the water stop.

At the intersections, volunteers cheered and blared car radios or rang cowbells. Feeling my arms swing and my weight shift, I found a rhythm. The meditative sway of my body calmed me, and the adrenaline made me glow. I may have looked like an overweight, middle-aged woman plodding through the suburban streets, but I felt like the T-shirt, "In my mind I'm a Kenyan."

I talked myself through the next hill. I frequently ran hills in my neighborhood. This was just another. But around the corner was a much larger hill, one I hadn't noticed when Ed and I had driven the course. My breath grew raspy. Again, I slowed, panting, lightheaded, and sad. "You're not a runner. You can't even run a 5k. Look at you in your silly T-shirt and expensive shoes. Who do you think you are?" Near tears, I let the voices roll across me. I watched the pavement pass beneath my feet. One step. Two steps. Three steps. Four.

When someone yelled, "Great job!" I barely looked. But a police officer leaning against the hood of her car caught my eye. I raised my head. I was almost up the hill! I waved and kept going.

At the top, several young children held cups of water. Two girls smiled while a little boy looked at the ground. I pushed toward him and slowed to look into his eyes. "Thank you!" I said, and he rewarded me with the tiniest smile.

Around the corner, we headed back toward the park and past the two-mile sign. Ahead was the giggling gaggle of girls, now walking. I remembered the y'chi (pronounced ee-chee) I'd learned in ChiRunning, and focused on the girls to pull myself down the road. I also imagined a bull's-eye on their backs with a rope attached to pull me toward them. The space between us slowly closed. Absorbed in each other's company, they didn't notice me passing them. For a moment, I remembered my niece giggling with her friends and I grew short of breath, but then remembered how brave she had been during the treatment. I was running in her honor.

Back at the park, I thanked the officer again. It seemed hours since that first runner had passed. I checked my watch, but I'd forgotten to start it. So much for fancy equipment.

With half a mile to go, I sped up. Relax and lean. Near the small library, I passed a woman with a stroller. Up a small incline and into the wooded area, I saw the "Beat Cancer" sign again. My breath came in gasps as I tearfully thought of Jamey. The finish line was to my right, but I didn't look. I passed the spot where Ed had been. Heart racing, I pumped my arms and legs. A runner ahead took a sharp right. I followed. The finish line lay just ahead. My heartbeat pumped in my ears. The large black clock read 42-something. Determined to beat 43:00, I swept past the clock, beneath the arch, and across the timing mats in 42:16. It felt like flying.

Ed hugged and kissed me. I hugged my friends and family who'd done the fun walk.

Exhausted and proud, I went to the shelter house for a banana and water, then back to the finish to wait for Krista. We watched people of all shapes, sizes, and abilities come in. The number of finishers dwindled. Still no Krista. I scanned the empty course and began to worry. In the weeks leading up to the race, she'd been having coordination problems due to a medication. The race crew was packing up.

I told them, "My friend hasn't finished." A man spoke into a walkie-talkie.

"The sweep car picked her up," he said.

A few minutes later, two volunteers helped her stumble across the finish line. She'd tried to run, but nearly collapsed on the big hill where the voices had almost stopped me. The kind police officer drove her to the finish. Later, a medication change would resolve the problem.

A group of us went to breakfast. Ecstatic and giggly with that floaty post-run glow, I relived each challenge I'd overcome as my friends and family listened. Maybe I was an athlete after all. Not only had I run despite the negative voices in my head, I'd run in public! I was strong, healthy, and famished.

***

At that first 5k, I fell in love with races. They're like a party on foot, complete with family, friends, food, running, and music (even if it's from car speakers). Plus, it fed my competitive side. Jogging past that pack of young girls—even though they were walking—made me happy I wasn't last. I would have preferred it if Krista hadn't been last, but was selfishly joyful it wasn't me.

Despite all this, the next day, I wandered the house moping. In the photos Ed had taken of our group and of me crossing the finish line, I thought I looked fat. No matter how much weight I lose, I still think I look fat. It bears little relationship to what I actually weigh.

"You haven't been this sad since you started running," Ed said, putting his arm around me. Blue, spent, and lost, I cried a lot. Seeing the children in wheelchairs or on crutches, many of them amputees like Jamey, had jolted me back to the five hundred days of her treatment and her untimely death. She should have been among the survivors. My heart ached with emptiness and longing.

I texted my sister, who was also re-experiencing her grief. While the race brought us together, it also stirred brutal memories. Jamey really was gone. I called Morgan and crawled into bed, where his warmth comforted me.

After two dark days spent mostly sleeping, I consulted the Penguins. Post-race doldrums were normal even when the race wasn't a memorial to a dead loved one. I'd been pushing for this goal for nearly six months and overcome my fear of running in public. Now it was over. The physical and psychological letdown reminded me of the first week in January, when everyone goes back to their post-holiday lives.

The Penguins knew the solution. "Sign up for another race!" I'd been so worried that I hadn't thought beyond that first 5k.

The internet revealed many options. The favorite was the Columbus Turkey Trot, a Thanksgiving morning race through the suburb where we live. It claimed to be "central Ohio's oldest and largest Thanksgiving Day tradition," around for nearly two decades. The race benefits Easter Seals, a charity I could support without heart-wrenching memories. I'd previously seen some of my friends at a local coffeehouse after they'd run it. At the time, I thought they were nuts, running on such a cold day. With my newfound love of racing, it seemed ideal.

Then my smile faded: five miles. I'd hoped for another 5k. I looked at the calendar. Nine and a half weeks until Thanksgiving. It had taken six months to train to run three miles. There was no way I could double that in nine and a half weeks.

I found a shorter race earlier in November but preferred to race on Thanksgiving Day. Another Thanksgiving race, a four-miler, still sounded too far, plus the giveaway was a bottle of wine. Not something I wanted. The Columbus Turkey Trot website featured photos of runners in turkey, pilgrim, and Native American costumes. *Runner's World Magazine* had voted it "Best Hometown Favorite." I sighed and closed the computer.

I brooded for another day, then remembered the "Ask the Coach" forum. There, as if someone had read my mind, the coach gave a woman who'd run her first 5k a nine-week schedule—exactly the number of weeks I had to train for a five-mile turkey trot! I swung from depression to hypomania—a mood shift that felt like a gift! I printed the schedule and asked Ed what he thought. He hugged me.

Ed, of all people, knows I need structure. This nine-week schedule would carry me beyond the 5k training to five miles. I didn't sign up but committed to training. I taped the printed schedule to the end of my bookcase, on top of the 5k plan, which was now history. Let the training begin!

CHAPTER 7

Fuse. Fuse. Fuse.

Before I ran the 5k, my MD sent word that I didn't have rheumatoid arthritis. Instead, I had the beginnings of a bone spur and the remnants of a prior sprained ankle that hadn't properly healed in high school. None of this explained my swollen ankle. She ordered an MRI.

Those claustrophobia-inducing devices, with their tunnels, loud magnets, and scary dye, petrify me. I made an appointment, then cancelled it. I made another appointment, then rescheduled it. Finally, over the phone, a woman at the lab reassured me I would only need to stick my ankle, not my whole body, into the machine. I drove myself and didn't ask for anti-anxiety medication.

In the waiting room, I did slow breathing and tried to distract myself from my heart palpitations and sweating palms by reading the women's magazines that littered the small tables. I stood several times to leave, but talked myself back into one of the vinyl chairs. In the prep interview, I asked about the dye and a woman in scrubs said it wouldn't be necessary. A wave of relief washed over me. Without the dye, I thought I would live through it. I again asked if my head would have to go into the machine. "Only your ankle," the woman confirmed.

Eventually, a different technician, a tall woman with dark hair and a furrowed brow, called me. I followed her into a locker room where she told me to remove my socks and shoes. Through an open door, the mouth of the giant machine gaped at me. I looked away. My hands shook as I put my socks and shoes in a locker. As I waited, I tried not to look, but my eyes were drawn to the dark central hole of the machine. I reminded myself that I didn't have to go in all the way.

The technician reviewed my medical information as I followed her into the MRI room. Her brusque tone and quick pace did nothing to reassure me. She secured my ankle in a boot and started rolling the bed into the gaping tunnel. My heart beat wildly. "Slow down!" I cried.

After a deep sigh, she agreed to inch me in with short bursts. Little by little, my legs went in. As my knees began to go in, I protested, "They said only my ankles!"

"They were wrong," she said, then gave me a number in centimeters which confused me.

"How much further?"

She sighed again and said, "Not far."

My heart beat in my throat and ears. I tried to breathe slowly. I hadn't asked to bring a paper bag. I clenched the washcloth she'd given me to put over my eyes. That made me even more claustrophobic, so I kept it in my sweaty hands.

As the machine continued, she handed me a pair of headphones. They blared country music, which I hate. She promised to switch to the smooth jazz station once she was in the control area for the test.

When I was in to my mid-thigh, she said "There we go," and turned to leave.

"Wait! Will I be able to talk to you?" I could almost hear her eyes roll as she reminded me there was a red button I could use to talk to her.

"Will that get me out?" I was afraid the device might swallow me completely while she was gone.

"No," she said. "We'll talk about whether you need to come out."

"Ready?" she asked. I could stall no longer. "Okay," I lied. The door closed.

A few seconds later, her voice came through the headphones. "I can't find smooth jazz." I suggested classical and a booming piano concerto, not soothing in the least, came through the headphones. I gritted my teeth. The music muted the loud magnets. She asked me to hold still for a few seconds, then to relax. She repeated this many times. The music changed and a softer song came on. After a few more times of my holding still and then relaxing, she said, "Let me make sure the images are okay." This was the longest wait. The classical music picked up tempo again and my breath and heartbeat grew louder in my ears. I couldn't take it and pressed the button.

"Yes?" she said.

"Are you coming?" I asked.

"In a minute," she said.

"Can you turn off the music?"

Finally, she spat me out of the dreadful machine. I started to sit up, but my foot was still restrained. She removed the plastic splint and said, "Sit up slowly. You might be lightheaded." I sat up and waited for my breathing to return to normal.

I felt grateful but silly. It hadn't been that bad. Once again, my mind had taken a trip it hadn't needed.

The technician met me in the interior lobby again. "Your doctor will have the results."

I thanked her and started to leave. She stopped me and said, "If you need another MRI, ask for an open MRI and anti-anxiety meds." Then she closed the door behind her.

***

A few days after the MRI, a letter from my primary care physician arrived: "Talocalcaneal coalition with osteoarthritis of the talonavicular joint, strain of syndesmotic and intrinsic ankle ligaments, and second metatarsal joint osteoarthritis. Next step is to see a foot and ankle surgeon."

Ten years before, both of my shoulders had frozen after I'd run a push lawn mower into a large rock. My primary care physician had referred me to a shoulder surgeon, who sent me to physical therapy. It took three rounds of PT sessions before I regained mobility in my arms but no surgery. I called the shoulder surgeon for a referral, since he didn't do ankles.

Still hesitant, I put off making the appointment. My family has a strange relationship to doctors. My mother had a ton of them and went frequently, but also consulted chiropractors and natural healers. She took supplements and went on food regimens, attempting to heal her chronic cough and, later, her arthritic pain. My father didn't go to the doctor unless he was gravely ill and ultimately waited too long to see the doctor who diagnosed his terminal cancer. Also, I'd been an attorney, and attorneys and doctors have had a love-hate relationship ever since the first medical malpractice case in history. I knew doctors wanted to help, but if you were a carpenter, everything looked like a nail.

Like my mother, I'd used natural techniques to treat chronic back pain. Egoscue Method "e-cises" kept me out of the back surgeon's office and I'd seen a chiropractor for my ankle, with limited success.

Still, my ankle continued to swell if I ran hard. It had swollen after the 5k. It hadn't puffed up, but it felt tight. After talking with Ed, chatting with the Penguins, and researching talocalcaneal coalitions, I went to see the surgeon.

I had written the appointment in my datebook, but an unsmiling woman at the front desk said I was there on the wrong day. I had to wait nearly an hour; the doctor wanted a different set of x-rays, and the office didn't have the right software to view the MRI file I'd brought.

Once the technician printed new films, a similarly unsmiling woman led me to a room. On the wall hung images of knee, ankle, and hip joints, and ads for pharmaceutical products. Heavy footsteps approached. The door opened to reveal a tall, heavyset man in a white coat that gaped in front. He entered, nearly filling the space between the wall and the table on which I sat. He roughly shook my hand, then picked up my slightly puffy ankle. He pressed his large fingers into the flesh around the bone and up and down my foot.

As he held my ankle, I cheerfully proclaimed, "I just ran my first 5k, and I'm training for a five-mile turkey trot!"

He released my foot from his fleshy grip and said, "Humans aren't built to run long distances." He told me how much he hated running. "I did a 5k once. Never again."

He explained that the bones in my ankle were too close together and just as matter-of-factly said, "We'll fuse it to avoid further deterioration."

"Did you look at the MRI?" He shook his head. "I have the radiologist's report. We'll do a full contrast MRI to get a better look." He touched my ankle bone. "If someone had caught this when you were a child, they could have fixed it." Then he added, "If you continue to run, it will ruin your ankles and knees."

My anger rose. I wanted to break something, but wouldn't get into a screaming match with a man six times my size.

"The girls up front will schedule the contrast MRI," he said and turned to leave.

I cleared my throat. "I'll think about it."

He turned back and glared. I focused on the anatomy posters.

After a few beats of silence, he said, "It will only get worse. In the meantime, you need to wear a leg brace and compression hose."

I said nothing. His stare felt like ice on the side of my head.

Finally, I faced him and said, "I want the x-rays and the records I brought."

"No," he said. "We'll keep them on file."

Now my voice rose, "I want them back and I want a copy of the new ones."

"Fine," he said, smirking. "The girls up front will handle the charges." Then he opened the door and pounded down the hallway. When the stomps ended, a door slammed.

In his wake, I sat on the bed and held my flushed face in my hands. Once I had calmed, I pulled the x-ray off the viewing box and took it with me. I might get a second opinion. I might not. Either way, this man wasn't coming near my ankle.

I fought with the grumpy front desk staff to get back the records I'd brought, even though the surgeon hadn't looked at them and I'd already paid for them elsewhere. To get a copy of the new x-rays, I had to go to another office across town and pay thirty dollars.

I took the prescription for compression hose and an ankle brace to the locally owned pharmacy in my neighborhood. A friendly woman pharmacist explained what they were. The stiff brace allowed no movement of the joint. I thought back to *Born to Run*, my research on minimalist shoes, and the ChiRunning classes. These concurred that when you support any joint, including the ankle, it weakens it by not allowing it to move as nature intended. I told her I didn't want the brace. The compression hose, though, seemed like a good idea. The pharmacist said she wore them on planes to prevent blood clots. I bought the hose.

At home, I cursed as I told Ed about the appointment. We talked about a second opinion, but feared the result would be the same. It had taken so much energy. I couldn't imagine doing it again.

***

The next day, I ran two slow, painful miles as the surgeon's words played a sadistic loop through my brain: Fuse. Fuse. Fuse. Fuse. Fuse. The dog, also sullen, lagged.

"What's up, pup?" I asked half-heartedly, but he wasn't talking. Could he hear my head?

My arms and legs swung more heavily the further I ran. Running, my new mood and self-esteem booster, would be stolen. I thought about lying down in the street. If I couldn't run, I wasn't sure I wanted to live. I was falling into a swirling mass of dread.

Before my appointment with the surgeon, I'd worn a knee brace Ed loaned me, which he'd had from a skiing accident, but it made no difference. I'd elevated or iced my ankle and the swelling went down, it but recurred each time I ran. I'd created rules: never run two days in a row or more than four days a week, and don't run hard. I researched shoes, form, and surfaces. I read, surfed the internet, and talked to other runners. But now, with the surgeon's words in my head, I'd have to give up.

Instead of running, I napped. Mr. Dawg's pleading eyes prompted me to walk the same distances we'd been running, but I wouldn't be able to complete the five miles necessary for the Turkey Trot, so I didn't sign up. This marked a new low.

At the end of September, when Ed and I went to a conference in Montreal, I meandered around the city in water shoes to strengthen my arches. I'd brought running gear but gave Ed excuses about not being used to running in urban areas. I didn't tell him the real reason. "Fuse. Fuse. Fuse." I thought about running on the health club treadmill. Even five minutes would help. But, stuck in the mental sludge, I couldn't face that either.

***

Back home from Montreal, I let a full week pass without running. Walking is excellent exercise, but it didn't give me the lift running did. Perhaps it would help if I walked faster, but I couldn't make myself do that either.

As the days passed, my energy level plummeted, and thoughts of parking the car in the closed garage with the motor running floated like clouds through my mind. I wrote about my mood and complained.

Ed asked why walking wasn't enough. I wasn't sure. Only the Penguins seemed to understand.

I researched "talocalcaneal coalitions" and found no cure. One writer said, "Sure you can run, as long as you can stand the pain." One study on resectioning the ankle cited a dismal success rate. It was commonly not diagnosed until it was too late to treat it. This compounded my poor mood.

Shortly after I'd received the original MRI report from my primary care physician, several weeks before my first 5k, and long before I'd seen the ankle surgeon, I'd emailed a renowned running doctor and asked him if it was okay to run with a talocalcaneal coalition. He'd said I wouldn't injure myself by running with the ankle condition and that minimalist shoes might help. It was then that Ed and I had tried to find minimalist shoes, with no luck, and I'd settled on water shoes.

But now, I doubted the running doctor. He hadn't seen my ankle, my x-rays, or the MRI report. He was probably just trying to hawk the minimalist shoes in his store. The longer I didn't run, the more I feared the surgeon might be right.

***

When I'd been running, the small goals and endocannabinoid flush gave me a daily boost. Without that, bleakness spread. I slept more and took the faithful dog for long, excruciatingly slow walks trying desperately to generate positive sensations. As we made our way through the neighborhood, I lamented my inability to run. My ankle was sore and puffy even though I wasn't running. I feared I'd permanently damaged it. Maybe even walking was off-limits. The dog didn't care. He walked, sniffed, peed, and trudged through leaf piles with his usual meditative concentration, no matter our pace. I wasn't sure if he was serene or indifferent.

Ed wrapped me in long hugs. He asked what the surgery entailed, which enraged me. I never intended to see that surgeon again. I appreciated the support from both man and dog, but it wasn't helping. My mood continued to plummet. I continued writing, trying to process my emotions, but my dark words pushed my mood lower and lower. I contemplated checking myself into the psych ward the way I had so many years before.

It wasn't just the lack of running. I'd lost ten pounds, but my weight had plateaued. Articles explaining that people who exercise sometimes gain weight seemed like a cruel joke. Running had lulled me into a false sense of entitlement. "I ran half a mile. I can eat what I want." Running, one of the most calorie-burning forms of exercise, doesn't burn that many. I'm slow. If I ran for half an hour, I might burn fifty calories, the number in a quarter of a bagel. I hadn't earned the whole bagel. You can't outrun your mouth.

A friend suggested I was gaining muscle. While muscle weighs more than fat and muscle cells do burn more calories than fat cells, there's a limit. Despite the exercise, I wore the same size pants, and they were tight. This was fat, not muscle. While exercising is better than not exercising, my workouts didn't justify extra food.

Despite having lost some weight, I still hated clothes shopping. Dressing room mirrors either make you look so much bigger than you are that you run home crying, or they make you look smaller, so you buy everything in sight and then cry at home because it all looks ugly in your bedroom mirror.

And let's not even mention my age. My birthday next August would put me at fifty, "over the hill." When I looked back, I lamented lost time and opportunities and wasted effort. Despite early years of success, I wasn't close to where I imagined being by fifty and had no idea how to get there. No books published. The weight battle continuing. My musculoskeletal health in jeopardy. I was talking myself into a death spiral.

Nearly drowning in these thoughts, I texted my sister, summarizing my self-recriminations as I wept at my desk. Then I immediately apologized. She, not I, had reason to be blue, losing her only child to cancer, but I sobbed anyway. I had thought running was a fountain of youth. I thought it would keep the weight off, prevent heart disease, stave off diabetes, and solve my mental health problems. Running had deluded me into thinking the dog and I were getting younger instead of aging. But even if running had been a cure, the doctors had snatched it away.

Every few days, I would almost give myself permission to run again. I'd tell myself to run slowly and not go far. At other times, I fumed at the surgeon. "Screw you! I will run again!" But each time, I'd succumb to the negativity, wipe away tears, and stomp around the house, pouting.

One night, crying so hard I could hardly breathe, I pounded on my keyboard. Painful emotions about being old, fat, and wounded rushed through my mind. I wept until my nose was snotty and my face wet. "Fuse, fuse, fuse, fuse, fuse," screamed my mind. I needed to accept my fate. Cried-out, I crawled into bed with Ed.

As I fell asleep, I began to dream...of running.

***

Eleven days after seeing the ankle surgeon, I saw my psychiatrist. The usually cheery lobby looked dim. The sound of the waterfall set my teeth on edge. By the time she called me in, I was sobbing.

"Tell me exactly what he said."

When I finished, she said, "Why don't you get a second…" then stopped. "Could you be a moderate runner?" She wondered if I could run less than my heart wanted, but not stop altogether. "It's not like you're going to run a marathon," she said. I had failed to mention my dream of a 26.2 sticker. For now, I just wanted to run five miles.

Like Ed and Mr. Dawg, my psychiatrist had watched my energy and sense of well-being improve. She believed running also prevented the need for a med increase. Usually she tampered with my med cocktail, but in the months I'd been running, the same dose worked. I still lacked focus, couldn't tolerate loud or unpredictable people, and was uber-sensitive to lights and noise, but, on the running days, I got out of bed. On those days, instead of sleeping until noon, I was up by ten and even showered.

She compared running to antidepressants. The drugs are hard on the kidneys and might kill me. People who take medications of any kind generally die earlier than people who don't. However, without them, I would probably die even earlier, by my own hand or in some accident I created. If I didn't die physically, I would die emotionally. Dead or in bed. It's a trade-off. I choose to take medications despite the possible consequences. Using the same logic, if I continued to run easy and enjoyed the benefits, but wound up crippled later, it would be better to run for as many years as possible and have a much better life.

As I left, she advised, "Find the best doctors you can, the innovators on the cutting edge." She had my attention. "Get a gait analysis. Seek physical therapy. Don't give up."

At home, before I sought the best doctors or did anything else, I pulled on my Lycra exercise pants, a T-shirt, and my fancy running socks, and, despite the articles I'd read about strengthening my feet, pulled on the cushioned Brooks Adrenaline running shoes. The dog glued himself to my side until I put on the leash. Sensing my excitement, he wagged his whole body, nearly knocking me down as we headed for the door. With my hand on the door handle, I wondered if I was risking permanent injury. But Morgan's ferocious tail wagging could mean only one thing: "Screw the ankle doc. Let's go!" The dog and the psychiatrist knew best. We headed outside.

It was a perfect sixty degrees, with the sun peeking out from the clouds. I started slowly. My ankle didn't hurt. My knee didn't hurt. I did my best to keep my pelvis tucked, my head up, and my knees slightly bent. From my earliest days running, and as confirmed by running in water shoes, the less I bounced, the happier were my ankle and knee. We trotted toward the ravine where we'd started six months before.

I didn't know about the future, but I knew what running was doing for me right now. I vowed to only seek medical advice from professionals who honored running. And I promised to trust myself. The dog held his tail high, barely increasing his gait to keep up with me. When his tail slapped my leg with a hearty thump, I thought my heart might burst. We were back!

CHAPTER 8

Turkey Trot

Five days after the dog and I snatched running from the pesky ankle surgeon's grip, we ran four miles—our longest run. October in Ohio means rustling leaves in a kaleidoscope of russet, scarlet, tangerine, and buttery yellow. I breathed the autumn air and focused on hip rotation, but forgot after a while. I relaxed into the aches and pains, letting the sensations float through my consciousness like clouds.

In our neighborhood, we rake leaves into the street in high, narrow piles the city collects. Morgan loves this, even though the piles are often more than one Labrador retriever tall. When I let Morgan tromp through one pile, he misjudged the depth, and I laughed while he flailed, righted himself, shook the leaves out of his stiff fur, then trudged on as if nothing had happened.

I wanted to emulate the dog's fluid stride and effortless serenity. I'd improved enough that Morgan now had to trot to keep up, but he did so with utter calm. No strain or bounce. His head and back remained level. Only his legs moved as he jogged smoothly along. His floppy ears didn't flop, and even his powerful hindquarters remained relaxed. His tail flagged aloft with a slight curve that made the blonde hairs at the tip blow in the breeze. Sometimes his tongue lolled, but even his panting was rhythmic.

Then, a woman with a border collie approached, and Morgan grumbled. I tried to move between him and the pair, but Morgan growled and stood on his hind legs, pulling me with him. When he let out a throaty, guttural bark, I pulled him back, hard. He stopped and looked back, tilting his head. "What do you want? I'm a dog."

Once the dog and woman were out of sight, he collected himself back into serene self-possession.

***

After each run, I wore the compression hose and propped my foot on the nearest chair to elevate it. I filled my online running log with "Way to go!" and "Atta girl!" I posted regularly in the Penguins forum about running moderately with safeguards to protect me from injury. I wanted to run into my nineties. In the forum, after running for just six months, I was an old-timer. Mentally, I thumbed my nose at the surgeon. If the word "fuse" came up in conversation, I reminded myself they were talking about electrical systems, not my ankle.

I remained confused. The surgeon told me not to run. The psychiatrist told me to be moderate. The renowned running doctor said I could run freely. Determined, I created another running formula. If my ankle swelled, I took a day off. I never ran two days in a row. I continued to apply ChiRunning principles (upright posture, easy lean, relaxed body, quick foot turnover) and didn't run fast.

Besides, pace is relative. Some people get faster over time. With my wonky ankle and the need to focus on form, my pace slowed. My ankle prevented me from throwing myself into running the way motivational articles suggested. In theory, I would get faster, but first I had to master efficiency. I slowed to keep my pelvis tilted and my head up. I picked up my feet, bent my knees, and imagined the world rolling along beneath me like a giant ball.

I was slow. I'd have to accept it.

I stopped taking ibuprofen to see how my ankle really was. It swelled, but not as much and not every time. When it became stiff and puffy, I didn't panic. I did not stop running.

***

A week later, on Saturday, I ran four and three-quarter miles with heavy legs and heavy breathing. Some days I thought I could run forever. I wished I'd never given up running years before and dreamed of running longer distances. Other days, I couldn't remember what had possessed me to run in the first place.

Today, the phrase "my sport is your sport's punishment" seemed apt. I didn't care about the gorgeous leaves or the automatic personal record (a "PR") since I'd never gone that far before. I didn't care that this was nearly the entire Turkey Trot distance. I wanted to quit.

Part of my unhappiness was being afraid to take Mr. Dawg that far. The weather was still warm, and dogs don't sweat so can easily overheat. I didn't want to carry water for both of us. I didn't even want to carry water for myself.

To deal with this, I'd mapped two 2.35-mile loops. After the first, I went inside, unhitched Morgan, went to the bathroom, drank water, then headed for the street to face the second lap alone on leaded legs. As I walked down the driveway, Morgan stood on the kitchen windowsill, barked, and whined. When I returned, Ed said he'd been inconsolable, pacing and whimpering the whole time I was gone. When I tried to pet him, he gave me the "How dare you?" look, which tired me even more.

October had been warm, so when the weather turned colder, my body hadn't acclimated. September had been hot and humid, and some folks at my first 5k had worn singlets, which I thought identified them as serious runners. The tank I'd worn wasn't a singlet, but it wasn't a T-shirt either, so I'd worn it proudly. As fall came, I had to find other clothes.

My favorite cold-weather running accessory was the soft, gray, cotton J. Crew hoodie I'd pulled from Jamey's closet when Amy told me to take what I wanted. The cuff was ripped, but it was the perfect layer. At twenty-nine degrees, I wore the hoodie over two long-sleeved cotton T-shirts, a neck gaiter, and gloves. I layered running pants over long johns and long socks. With Jamey's hood up and her memory in my heart, I didn't notice the wind.

The Penguins told me about the *Runner's World* "What to Wear" calculator, but it was designed for people fast enough to break a sweat in the first ten minutes. Not me. I added a layer at their suggestion. The general rule is to dress as if it is twenty degrees warmer. I calculated it to ten degrees. Plus, I'd rather be sweaty at the end than cold at the beginning.

***

Two weeks before the Turkey Trot, I challenged myself to run five miles (the distance of the Turkey Trot) without the dog. To the average person, the difference between 4.7 miles and 5 miles is "point three" miles. To me, it was the width of the Grand Canyon. I expected to have a heart attack, trip and fall, or to collapse mid-run far from our house, unable to walk home. I didn't yet carry my phone, so couldn't call Ed. Besides, I usually ran during the day when most people, including him, were at work. I couldn't even nap on someone's lawn until they noticed.

The mental part of longer runs also frightened me. Even though I'd been meditating since my early thirties and my husband and I regularly attended ten-day silent retreats, I feared boredom. To most people, retreats sound like the epitome of boredom. Sit for forty-five minutes. Walk for thirty minutes. Sit for forty-five minutes. Eat a meal. Repeat three times a day for ten days, interrupted only by an evening lecture. You'd think adding less than half a mile to a run wouldn't scare me. But I was uncertain where the limit of my tolerance for boredom ended. Five miles might make me snap.

That day, the second mile was the most difficult. This is typical. About one-third of the way through a run, my mind says I'll never make it. But that day I learned, and have relearned repeatedly since, if I keep running, it gets better. When I finished the third mile, the inner glow started. At the end of mile four, my feet felt lighter and my pace quickened. When our house came into view at mile five, I was ecstatic.

Inside, I scratched the pouting dog's ears, went online, and signed up for the Columbus Turkey Trot.

***

When I picked up my packet for the Turkey Trot, Barry, one of the more "mature" staffers at the running store, warned that the first downhill mile might trick me. "Save something for the end. You'll need to run that mile back up." I thanked him and took the long-sleeved orange tech shirt that had a child's handprint turkey drawing emblazoned on the front.

But I'd come down with a cold. The Penguins said I could run if the cold was from the "neck up." If it was in my chest, I shouldn't. I had the sniffles and sometimes coughed, but thought it was post-nasal drip. I sat on the side of my bed, examining myself. My chest didn't feel heavy until I breathed in and out a few times. Then it felt heavy, but it always felt heavy when I paid attention. I asked Ed to listen to me breathe. "You're fine," he said. "Run." I wanted to agree, but that meant I had to run five miles in public. I scanned the training logs. I'd put in the miles. I listened to my breathing again. It sounded raspy, but that was normal when I was freaking myself out.

***

What Barry hadn't warned me about was parking. With nearly four thousand people registered, parking places on the streets three blocks from the shopping center where the race was to start were full. Undeterred, Ed pulled into an "ambulance only" space and we argued about who would pay the towing fee ("It's your race." "It's your car!").

With half an hour to go, part of me wanted to stay in the warm car, but another wanted to find the start. I kissed Ed and joined the milling crowd. Even layered up, I shivered.

Headed for the inflatable arch, I dodged a man and woman wearing aprons, a pair of standard poodles in costume (the black one a pilgrim, the brown an Indian), a family, each member of which wore a stuffed "stuffed" turkey on his or her head, someone dressed head-to-toe as a turkey, complete with wattle, and many others in pilgrim hats and Indian headbands.

A fine mist fell and I could see my breath. Runners stood in clumps, talking and stomping their feet to stay warm. I couldn't find the friends I knew were also running. Ed was out there somewhere, but we hadn't planned to meet until the finish. Cold and awkward, I didn't feel like striking up a conversation with random strangers. Eventually, the horn sounded and our throng headed down Lane Avenue.

Just as Barry predicted, I sped down that first downhill, then sagged. But I turned a corner on the Ohio State University campus and there stood Ed, holding a bottle of water. The night before, he had pored over the course map with a highlighter, figuring out how to meet me despite the closed streets. I didn't know there would be aid stations.

Seeing Ed revived me. I sped up. Outside Ohio Stadium, I caught Doug, my ChiRunning instructor. He was ChiWalking as fast as I was running. We chatted. I was no longer cold.

He pulled ahead, leaving me alone to lament my heavy legs and tired feet. When a woman about my age said aloud to no one, "This is where they need porta potties." I replied, "Or a Depends station." She giggled.

As we passed the mile four marker, she cheered. "One more mile!" But I could see the long hill ahead. Undaunted, she continued to chatter, confiding that she was a breast cancer survivor. "My son-in-law better be fast enough to get a pumpkin pie!" We wouldn't be among the first two thousand finishers to get one.

Our talk slowed and our breathing grew ragged as we climbed until we crossed the line together. Ed took a picture of us all, with her holding the pie her son-in-law had won. On the ride home, the after-run glow warmed me as much as the car heater.

At Thanksgiving with my family, my sister teased that running justified all the calories. That voice inside me growled, "Running won't fix everything." I told it to shut up and continued to eat.

***

While I collected race bibs, Ed earned accolades of his own. Back in October, *Columbus Monthly Magazine* had awarded him one of their coveted "CFO of the Year" awards for his work as Chief Financial Officer at House of Hope for Alcoholics, a long-term residential treatment facility. On any given day at this tiny nonprofit, Ed could be found doing anything from balancing the books to writing grants. He also led conflict resolution workshops and sometimes fixed the plumbing in the two Victorian mansions that housed the center. Ed had joined the agency when it was in financial trouble and turned it around. I liked to think of him as a knight on a white horse. The *Columbus Dispatch* interview article featured a dashing photo of him wearing a suit and tie while standing in the commercial kitchen remodeled with funding he acquired.

In December, Ed received a second honor when the Humanist Community of Central Ohio (HCCO) awarded him their coveted Humanist of the Year Award. He served on the HCCO board and was active in numerous good Samaritan activities, ranging from "bleed and feed" (a monthly blood drive) to the group's Adopt-A-Highway project. In a sweet role reversal, I proudly stood on the sidelines at the award ceremonies as he gave acceptance speeches and was recognized for his hard work, intelligence, and big heart.

I'd swung from anxiety at being seen running at all, to manic excitement at toeing the line, and sweet exhaustion mixed with a sense of accomplishment at the finish. I also loved swag. What's not to love about a Christmas-themed sweatshirt two sizes too big (my mistake for underestimating my weight loss), and yet another coffee mug when I already had boxes full in the basement? I could be addicted to worse things. To finish 2011, I ran two more 5ks: "Snowflake 5k" and "Running in the New Year."

When snow fell at the Snowflake 5k, I wondered if that made me a real runner. I used ChiRunning principles to "relax and lean" enough to chase down a woman at the finish. When I made the mistake of thanking her for helping me run faster, she scowled and replied, "Thanks for kicking my ass!" Oops.

On the afternoon of New Year's Eve, I wore the long-sleeved Turkey Trot technical shirt at "Running in the New Year." No more cotton next to my skin. The forty entrants in the church parking lot looked fit and fast. I wanted to leave, but Ed had driven half an hour to get us there. He read my thoughts. "So what if you come in last?"

Before I could argue, the race director yelled into a bullhorn for us to line up. I tried to step behind the last couple, but the man refused. "My wife thinks she'll be last." He pointed to a woman in a pink hoodie. Next to them stood an older man carrying a toddler on his shoulders.

The race began, and the couple passed me before we left the parking lot. On the main street, a car honked and swerved as a nonchalant policeman watched. He casually pointed across the street toward a river trail where I could see the woman in the pink hoodie.

The excitement of starting and nearly being plowed down by a car had distracted me, but now the desolate expanse of scrub tree lines and empty fields left room for negative mind chatter. "Old. Fat. Slow." If I could just keep the pink hoodie in sight, like a small security blanket.

When the woman slowed to a walk, I grew close enough to make out the folds in her hood. As I approached, she turned, gave me a determined look, started running, and pulled away.

A creek wound along the wooded trail. Except for an occasional car, it was quiet. The distance between the woman and me continued to increase until I lost sight of her. Trying to enjoy the run, I smelled the crisp air, took in the dark gray tree trunks and the occasional green foliage winter hadn't frozen.

I crossed a few streets, and then a couple walking a dog came from the opposite direction. I looked behind me for the man with the boy on his shoulders, but he wasn't there. I circled back to the next street. Halfway up a small hill, I saw the woman in the pink hoodie again... walking. She picked up her pace, but without energy. I passed her easily, embarrassed by my pride.

I ran harder, worried the pink hoodie woman might catch me. I caught the elderly man with the child still on his shoulders. "We took a little shortcut," he said as I passed. It had never occurred to me that someone would cut the course.

A handful of people cheered as I crossed into the parking lot where Ed was waiting. I joined him and the small crowd to watch for the others.

The man shouldering the child slow-jogged past as we yelled and clapped. Close behind, the woman in the pink hoodie jogged in. We hollered, whistled, and cheered as if she were the lead runner.

My cheeks burned. I'd been out to win even if winning meant beating only a grandfather carrying his grandson and a woman in a pink hoodie. They helped me set a new personal 5k record, but I had learned not to thank them.

Ed took a photo of me lying on a park bench, as if I had collapsed, to post on Facebook. This was the new me. I'd gone from lying on the sofa to "Running in the New Year."

That night, we watched television with friends as the ball dropped. Headed into the cold of January, I wondered how I would manage to not quit this thing I'd grown to love. I pushed the thoughts out of my mind, toasted my friends, and kissed my husband.

CHAPTER 9

The Land of Enchantment

This wasn't the first time I'd chased down a dream. In 1997, I convinced Ed we should move to Taos, New Mexico. We had only been married four years. I'd attended three week-long workshops with bestselling author Natalie Goldberg and had convinced myself that attending every workshop she offered would teach me to write a book. Certain the New Mexico sunshine and art would also give me a new outlook on life, I told everyone who would listen. We put our Ohio house on the market, and it sold in three days.

In Taos, on a July day, Ed and I sat outside in the sunshine in front of our realtor's office. A white Subaru Outback pulled into a space in front of the copy shop next door. I immediately recognized the dark-haired woman behind the wheel—Natalie. She climbed out carrying several file folders, saw us, then stared.

It took a minute for me to muster the courage to say, "Hi, Natalie."

"Are you visiting?" she asked.

"No," I beamed. "We're moving here."

Her dark eyes grew suspicious, but she asked about the location of our new house and invited us to meet at the library to talk the next day. Then she went into the copy shop.

I only remember one thing from our conversation at the library. "Taos is wild, you know," she repeated. I had grown up on a fifty-acre farm in rural Ohio. We'd raised cattle, soybeans, and corn. I'd shoveled horse manure and baled hay. I thought I knew "wild." If she was attempting to dissuade us, it did no good. Two months later, Ed and I were living on the mesa in a house with a stunning view of Taos Mountain.

***

At Natalie's workshops, I sat with nearly sixty others in rows of folding chairs in the adobe-style conference building at Mabel Dodge Luhan House, straining to absorb her every word. Natalie coined the term "writing practice" in her best-selling book *Writing Down the Bones*, which blended writing with Zen principles. Her mix of Buddhism and creativity suited my meditation practice.

The universal principles she taught extended far beyond writing. In her primary "rule of writing practice," she commanded us to, "Keep your hand moving." The creative mind and the inner critic for which she used the Zen term "monkey mind," tangle together and form a stranglehold on expression. To free the creative energy, you must "keep your hand moving." Trudging was a good thing. Natalie's admonitions to "Continue under all circumstances" and "Don't be tossed away," edicts handed down by her Zen teacher, Katagiri Roshi, also applied to more than writing. I was already applying this on days when getting out of bed was half the battle.

In the workshops, we wrote ten-minute pieces in spiral notebooks about everything from "mashed potatoes" to "your biggest regret." Don't like the topic? No matter. Write anyway. Pain in your legs from sitting in a folding chair for five days? Not to worry. "Don't be tossed away." Again, I quickly saw the parallels between writing and living with depression. Years later, I would see how these principles applied to running as well.

***

In addition to these principles, I gained a community of writers who shared similar goals. Women like me, mostly in their thirties or forties, attended the workshops. We meditated, did slow walking, and wrote. Stories of hardship and joy poured from our pens, and then we read aloud with no comment. Natalie divided us into small groups, and we spent hours writing and reading aloud while sitting in Adirondack chairs on the sandstone pavers that surrounded the main building. Cottonwoods stretched above us, swaying in the breeze.

Living in Taos, I did not have to pay for travel or lodging, so attended all four of Natalie's workshops each year. The magical week of the workshop brought energy and confidence. I pushed through, much like I had for years while practicing law. But once the workshop finished and my fifty-nine friends left for their mostly out-of-state homes, I was alone again with my suffering. Ed did his best to support me emotionally, but at one point he was working three jobs to make what he had easily earned at one job back in Ohio.

After we'd moved to Taos, Michele, Natalie's partner at that time, suggested we form a writing practice group to meet between workshops. I posted flyers at the library and in several coffee shops, and soon six of us were meeting once a week to write and read aloud in a coffee shop. While this filled some of the space between workshops, I only wrote when I was with the group. When I was alone in our lovely mesa home, I could not face the empty page.

***

Ed and I had hosted Michele and Natalie for lunch at our house the first month we arrived. Thanks to the writing group, Michele was becoming a good friend, but outside of the workshops, Natalie kept her distance. I knew she needed privacy but was desperate to learn as much from her as possible.

After six months, Natalie called to invite me to meet for tea at a coffeehouse on the north side of town. Here she admitted she had been "keeping an eye on me."

"So many people want a piece of me," she said. "I needed to make sure you weren't some crazy stalker."

I couldn't blame her. I was a bit obsessive.

Apparently reassured, Nat invited me to meet her once a week to talk about writing. At those meetings, she read a few of my pieces and offered suggestions, but mostly told me to continue doing writing practice. "You have to write a lot to figure out what you really want to write about." I found this discouraging, but knew it was true.

She also invited me to a writing group at her home. We met once a week in a zendo room she'd created at her Earthship house.

Built from aluminum cans and dirt, it sat wedged into a hillside. Big windows opened to a view of the mesa and the enormous sky. We sat in silence, then walked in silence, before settling down to write twenty-minute pieces we then read aloud. Most of the others knew each other. That didn't matter. We continued under all circumstances.

Eventually, she asked me to assist her at the workshops. I spent twenty minutes teaching the basic rules of writing practice to the large group and rang the bell at the walking and sitting sessions, while she met with small groups of participants. I also met with individuals who were having trouble dealing with the overwhelm that sometimes comes from diving so deep into writing. I related to their intense emotions. Honored to help Natalie, I needed the structure the role provided when often, even in the workshops, I felt untethered.

***

A year after Ed and I arrived, Natalie moved to Minnesota to study Zen. She kept her Earthship on the mesa and we continued the sitting, walking, and writing group in her absence, but except for workshops, I rarely saw her.

Meanwhile, prompted by the knowledge that prescription antidepressants cause weight gain, I quit taking my antidepressants and tried some "natural" remedies with disastrous results. Suicidal, I considered hospitalization, but the nearest psych ward was in Santa Fe, an hour and a half drive down the two-lane road through the Rio Grande Gorge. Convinced Ed would die in a car crash if he had to make that drive every day, I refused the hospital. Instead, Ed and I arranged for friends to check on me hourly. Ed already drove to Santa Fe once a week for a mediation certificate course. I insisted on riding along so that, when the car crashed, I would perish with him. Ed doubted we would crash or die but enjoyed the company. During his classes, I found a coffeehouse and wrote about my misery.

Eventually, I went back on meds. The suicidal ideation passed, but the episode left me hollow and exhausted.

Plus, the magic of "The Land of Enchantment," as people call New Mexico, didn't capture me. Much as I tried to find a home there, and, even though I now had two writing groups to spend time with between workshops and had found the recovery community, Taos left me uncomfortable. As Natalie had promised, Taos was wild, unkempt, disorderly, sometimes violent, and unfamiliar. I hadn't experienced this level of wildness in Ohio and hadn't recognized it in my short visits. To others, northern New Mexico is a great adventure, a needed shake-up, relief from the boredom of other parts of the country. But my shaky mental health required stability, familiarity, and order.

Ed adapted to Taos much better than I did, but my welfare concerned him. He agreed we should leave. Born and raised in Los Angeles, he went to school at Berkeley and might have liked to head to California. But he understood my need to go home. By March 2000, we had moved back to Ohio and were living in the suburban neighborhood through which I would eventually carry a digital timer to chase yet another dream.

CHAPTER 10

Structure

Despite the familiarity of home, dark Ohio days ushered in slippery black moods. I'd found running, and it brought temporary relief, energy, and even joy, but part of me still wished I could disappear. In late December, a Penguin announced the Hundred Days Challenge. The goal was to move for thirty minutes each day for the first hundred days of 2011. I already exercised several days a week. Perhaps a daily routine would stave off the winter spiral.

I had never exercised for thirty minutes every day. Growing up on a farm, I baled hay and shoveled manure. I ran from the house to the barn or cantered through the woods pretending to be a horse, but my first love had been music, not sports, and especially not gym class. During softball, the gym teacher sent uncoordinated band geeks like me to the outfield, hoping no one would hit the ball to us. Dodgeball terrified me. Boys and girls alike hurled the red rubber ball at me, hard, for an easy out. On the bleachers, I stung with red marks on my body and shame in my heart at being so afraid while my classmates thrived. Even though I loved school, I'd feign illness to avoid the humiliation of forced exercise.

In the Hundred Days Challenge, I got to choose. I could hop, skip, jump up and down, do yoga, stretch, or roll on the floor. Any movement counted. I liked the potential for variety. The structure and online community might help me stay active.

Depression, PTSD, and bipolar disorder suppress my internal motivation. Overthinking turns decision-making into paralysis. Faced with too many choices, I fixate on weighing the options. Perfectionism, fear of failure, and certainty that any task is too difficult leave me overwhelmed. I'm more likely to do something someone else suggests.

Some days, even putting on exercise clothes was too much. I broke it into tiny steps. First, walk to the shoe rack. But then I had to decide which pair. Once I selected a pair, I sat down to put them on. But before that came the question of socks. Thick or thin? And what color? I had a drawer full by now. The same was true of other clothing. How many layers? Which ones? All this made for potential paralysis.

A running schedule and the structure of the Hundred Days Challenge helped. These weren't completely external because I'd chosen them, but the printed schedule taped to the end of my bookcase acted as something outside myself and removed the decision on how far or what days. To remove the quandary of where to run, I developed a series of routes. I chose a route of the mileage specified for that day and was off. Well, after choosing socks, clothes, and shoes. Plus, there was the watch to put on and the dog to leash, but eventually I headed out the door.

***

Prompted by the Hundred Days Challenge, in January, I did what all good New Year's Resolutioners do. I joined a gym, intent on lifting weights. In my younger days, when I'd run solely to lose weight, I'd lifted weights as compulsively as I'd run, developing defined arms and legs. I doubted I'd achieve that kind of physique twenty years later but was all for transforming a little flab.

McConnell Heart Health Center, fifteen minutes from our house, is bright, shiny, well-maintained, and caters to cardiac rehab patients. The weight machines remember your settings. I didn't have to carry a clipboard or rely on my ever-failing memory. And the locker room has fluffy towels.

For a gym, it's quiet. I can't abide loud noises. Sound vibrates in my head and against my skin. In large stores, squeaking shopping cart wheels and squawking loudspeakers sometimes force me into the bathroom to sit for a few minutes before I can shop. At McConnell, machines still clanked and treadmill motors hummed over light rock, but it happily lacked the high-volume stereo, the grunting body builders, and the women laughing in high-pitched squeals. The muffled sounds didn't hurt. While the volunteers and staff insisted on saying hello, which I found challenging, I could get used to that. It was desensitization.

I also liked the lack of gym bunnies. During the day, members were gray-haired men and women in loose-fitting shorts and T-shirts, with the occasional person younger than sixty. They moved slowly and quietly, wore no Lycra, spandex, push-up bras, or ripped tank tops. The most form-fitting thing I'd seen was yoga pants. Even the bathing suits were modest. Comfortable in my boot-cut gym pants and cotton T-shirts, I wasn't the only one with bed head and no makeup. It was nice to be a younger member. Was that grandfather checking me out? All the better.

Another draw to joining a gym was my fear of falling. In winter, fluffy mounds of snow, cutting winds, and freezing rain turn the central Ohio streets to ice. I wasn't ready to buy Yaktraks and slip down the streets. I became a regular on the indoor track, running in circles above the gym, where I watched the Medicare set work the weight machines below. I counted laps on my fingers and prided myself on running several miles at a time.

Mr. Dawg, who didn't appreciate my gym participation, gave me the sad eyes when I left the house in workout clothes without him. He pouted upon my return. But the salt and cinders used to maintain the roads might harm his paws, so I left him at home.

***

For accountability during the Hundred Days Challenge, participants posted daily activities on social media. I loved posting my wide variety of activities, even including snow shoveling and snow blowing (harder than it looks).

The gym had a half basketball court, so one day I shot baskets. My arms were weak, and at first I barely reached the basket. Within ten minutes, I was hitting the backboard. I'd played basketball only when required in middle school. Now, more than thirty years later, grade school friends cheered my achievement online.

I also used the two pools. The warm-water pool was like an enormous bath tub with jets. I took water movement classes and had difficulty keeping up with white-haired ladies twenty years my senior, but they asked me to come back. With sky, snow, and trees monochrome, the steamy blue water soothed my joints and mind.

At first, I found the Olympic-size lap pool intimidating, but a few orientation classes with a trainer helped. I did half-hour sessions of water-walking exercises, which were also more difficult than they looked.

On other days, I stayed home, tuned to an '80s station, and jitterbugged, twisted, or two-stepped around the living room. The confused dog barked and jumped at me. When I refused to cease, he lay down in a corner with his back turned and feigned sleep.

Rope jumping also turned out to be difficult. One thirty-minute session of bouncing on the hardwood floors did nothing for my unhappy ankle, which swelled and hurt the next day.

One snowy day, I walked up and down the single flight of stairs from our kitchen to the basement. After ten minutes, I needed to sit down. I did stretchy-band exercises and yoga to finish the session.

I'd printed a Hundred Days Challenge chart and stuck a sticker on the appropriate square each day. It made the winter months pass more easily and helped my self-esteem. Some online friends applauded my efforts. Others probably found it annoying, but no one criticized me directly. Given my newfound love for exercise, I might have unfriended them.

***

At McConnell, I skipped the treadmills in favor of the indoor track. I'm afraid of flying off the back or getting stuck in the treadmill belt and flying around like George Jetson and his dog, Astro. The whirring and vibration hurt my teeth and, when I stepped off, I was dizzy.

There's also the peril of standing next to someone who is "obviously" watching. Yes, I'm paranoid, but that doesn't mean she's not looking at me. Plus, it's boring to stand in one place on the "dreadmill" as the Penguins called them. You can watch television, but we haven't had one since 1996. And I always wind up stationed in front of the television tuned to a reality show where people covered in spiders eat live worms.

I might have enjoyed the precise measurement of my heart rate, mileage, and pace or the variety offered by the treadmill's hill and interval workouts. Instead, I preferred the hills in my neighborhood. For intervals, I speed up and slow down. Maybe, if we had a treadmill in our basement where I could watch a documentary or listen to an audiobook without being seen, I might enjoy it. Maybe I haven't spent enough time on treadmills. Perhaps I would hone the ability to stay upright while being jettisoned backward. Or maybe I just hate treadmills.

I only headed for McConnell if snow or ice covered the streets. I preferred running outdoors. Icicles on my eyelashes and a few flakes of snow in my hair made me feel like a badass. Our neighborhood has excellent public services, including what a friend jokingly calls "horizontal snow plows." They practically catch the flakes before they hit the ground. Only in a severe storm have the streets remained unplowed for more than a day.

On one such bitter day, I headed to the third-floor track. The wall of high windows overlooking the lake and woods provided a view of leafless tree tops and the steel gray sky. Across the track, a gray-haired man with a gaunt face moved in the fluid yet rhythmic motions of a race walker. I envied the clicker he held to count laps, since I often lost track counting on my fingers. I jogged around the first lap to get warmed up, then picked up speed. A few times around, I realized he was lapping me, not by much, but walking faster than I was running. Over time, I would see him regularly on the track and later at races, always friendly and determined. Being a back-of-the-packer, I needed to get used to this. Still, it hurt my pride a little. Okay. A lot.

Colder weather required more layers. One day, when it was in the low thirties with bright sun and no cloud cover to hold heat in, wind chill made it seem like the mid-twenties. I pulled a long-sleeved cotton T-shirt over a cotton short-sleeved T-shirt and topped that with

Jamey's cotton hoodie. I added a neck gaiter with a built-in double screen that heats your breath as it comes through, white gloves with tiny metal fibers woven in to conduct heat from my skin, and black wrap-around sunglasses. I looked like a cross between Michael Jackson and Darth Vader.

The dog had his fur. He was fine.

Half a mile in, as we jogged back up the ravine hill into the neighborhood, my face was sweating. I pushed down the gaiter. The frost-covered lawns were still green, but a subtler hue than in summer and grass blades peeked through. The dog jogged steadily beside me unfazed. After the first mile, my back dripped with sweat. How much nicer it was to be warm. I turned the corner to a street with wider lots. The wind blowing across the open yards between houses began to freeze my sweat-soaked cotton layers. Shivering, I now understood the phrase, "cotton kills." My cotton shirt froze to my skin like a wet tongue on a metal pole. I'd have to thaw out before I undressed. My teeth chattered as I envied Mr. Dawg's thick coat. At home, once I was warm enough to peel off the layers, I hopped into a lukewarm shower. A hot one would have burned.

The Penguins pointed me toward technical fabrics like the shirt from the Turkey Trot. "Layers and NO cotton!" On our next run, I wore tech shirts and long synthetic underwear under synthetic pants. I was cold at the start, but not frozen at the finish. I felt die-hard and happy.

CHAPTER 11

Endurance Athlete

Back in mid-November, before the Turkey Trot, I told my primary care physician I was unwilling to have my ankle fused. She understood, but cautioned, "The ankle joint will only take so much." My primary care physician had a foot injury that made it impossible for her to run. She, like the ankle surgeon, didn't appreciate the benefits of running. I asked her for a referral to physical therapy and said, "I'd like a runner."

Andrew, the physical therapist at Ohio State, prescribed balance and stretchy-band exercises. At the end of each session, he wrapped a bag of ice to my ankle. It always hurt at first, but only for a minute. Andrew, also a runner, didn't think running would do more damage, even though my left ankle would never have the same range of motion as the right. After eight sessions, my ankle had more range of motion and withstood more weight. It still swelled when I ran, but not as much, and, when I did the exercises, my knee didn't hurt.

To analyze my stride, Andrew videotaped me on a treadmill. I doubted this accurately reflected my gait since I was afraid of the horrendous machine. He took footage from both the side and back, which we reviewed. Not coincidentally, I was collapsing on the left side since my wonky ankle didn't bend enough. Instead, my knee did the bending. He suggested I run with my feet farther apart. I tried this for a few runs, but it was awkward and didn't seem to change anything.

I'd hoped for an examination similar to that performed by the Running Injury Clinic in Calgary, Alberta, Canada, leaders in 3-D gait analysis. At the time, Ohio State had nothing that sophisticated. Running injuries typically fall into just a few classes, so the same sets of exercises remedy most injuries. I printed the most applicable exercises, primarily targeting the adductor and abductor thigh muscles, and did those along with the ones Andrew gave me. I used the wobble boards and stretchy bands at the gym to continue physical therapy long after my insurance no longer paid. Again, there was no huge difference, but keeping the ankle moving helped. This proved the phrase my elderly uncle, the former runner, used as his signature: "Don't rust!"

Seeing Andrew boosted my confidence. One day, as I refused to quit after falling off the wobble board several times, he said, "You endurance athletes sure are tenacious." Endurance athlete! I floated out of the clinic.

Time would tell if I was in denial about my ankle. I only listened to what I wanted to hear. It's not uncommon for me to think I'm an exception. While my primary care doctor hadn't said not to run, like the surgeon, she believed running would do harm. So here I was going against the advice of two MDs. Perhaps ignoring my doctors' orders was stubbornness. Perhaps it was mental illness. The running doctor, my therapist, psychiatrist, physical therapist, husband, dog, and Penguin friends, all encouraged me to keep running. Perhaps they were thinking short-term, but they didn't want me to stop. My psychiatrist had told me to be a moderate runner, but I'm not sure moderate is in my vocabulary. I said, "Ankle be damned" and continued.

***

In March, Leslee, a friend from Louisville who was also doing the Hundred Days Challenge, suggested I try a bigger race. She'd run a half marathon before and was training again. Columbus hosts the Capital City Half Marathon every spring, which includes a "quarter marathon" of 6.55 miles. Despite my nightmares about getting lost in the crowd or veering off course at this huge race, Leslee promised it would be fun, so I signed up. Then I went online and found a training schedule.

***

In late April, we traveled to Des Moines, Iowa where Ed attended a humanist conference. While he was in the workshops, I mapped a six-mile run, as training for the slightly longer Cap City Quarter. I cut the paper map I'd printed in the hotel business center into a small square to carry. With Mr. Dawg at the kennel, this would be my longest solo run.

The Des Moines River, a formidable tributary of the Mississippi, divides the town with numerous bridges spanning the river. I ran parallel to the river for a block before I saw the long, red pedestrian bridge my map directed me to cross. The overhead steel beams spooked me, and I froze.

I don't like driving or even walking over bridges, but there was no other way to follow the route. The bridge wasn't likely to collapse, but I can't swim, and the dark waters below threatened. The bridge wasn't high, but it looked long—three or four hundred feet across. I stared at it. It stared back. I missed the dog.

I considered returning to the hotel to nap. Ed would be in meetings. I pushed the thought aside. Giving in would only make things worse.

A few years before I started this training, during a stint when I'd stopped taking my meds, I began having panic attacks again, especially on the freeway. I was fine if I drove in the right lane. Driving at night also brought them on. I stopped going to evening activities. Each time I pulled out of our driveway, I felt a tug on my heart, as if it something had tied it to our house. The tie stretched and stretched as I drove, threatening to snap. My world grew smaller and smaller, until the attacks also began at home. More than once, Ed brought me a paper bag and chamomile tea while I sat on the edge of the bed, gasping.

I went back on medication but knew the true remedy. I had to do what scared me, or the anxiety would build. Once I pushed through, the fear receded.

Staring at the bridge, I remembered those anxious nights, adrenaline surging through my veins. I remembered those days on the freeway, breathing into a paper bag. I remembered exit ramps and highway berms and the screaming in my head. I thought of the small bridge that crosses the little creek at home. If I didn't cross this bridge, I might be afraid to run over that tiny bridge, or eventually even near a river. And one day, I wouldn't be able to run at all.

I glared back at the bridge. It glared back. I chose a spot on a brick building on the opposite shore as a focal point and took off. My heart pounded and my mind screamed, "Turn back!" It seemed a force from behind was pulling me backward. I strained against it and flew past the red beams, certain my heart would explode. Halfway across, as the building on the other side grew closer, the mental screaming stopped. On the sidewalk near the street, I walked to catch my breath. I'd have to run back across later but would literally cross that bridge when I came to it. For another fifteen minutes, I shuffled along, barely noticing the city. That bridge had taken it out of me. Sometimes when I face a challenge, my confidence grows. Today, it had drained me.

Ahead, where the Des Moines meets the Red River, loomed another bridge. When I'd seen it on the map, I'd hoped for a wide and low vehicle bridge, beneath which I couldn't see the dark water. But this was a converted railroad bridge, longer than the previous one. As a cyclist passed me, then crossed the bridge, the wooden slats rattled, sending a shiver down my spine.

There would be consequences if I didn't cross, but I couldn't summon the energy. Someone else might find its rusting beams and wooden planks beautiful, but I found no beauty in it. When a second bicyclist wobbled across, rattling not only the bridge but also my spirits, I turned. I'd exceeded my limit of scary bridge crossings for that day. Resigned, I ran back the way I'd come.

I wound my way back to the walking bridge which I intended to master. I'd desensitized myself by repeating frightening things in small doses. As they become familiar, they are less terrifying.

My heart still pounded hard as I thought of the water below, but I went onto the bridge anyway. A family stood fearlessly, halfway across. Unlike the wooden bridge, this bridge didn't rattle. It bounced but made no sound. I reminded myself that I'd done this before. But having done a thing doesn't always help, since panic attacks function at the illogical, earthworm level of the brain. This time, however, repetition worked. I waved to the family as I passed, aware that they were oblivious to how huge this accomplishment was for me. On the other side, breathless and ecstatic, I focused on where to run next, since I hadn't followed my route. Up a long hill sat the capital building. I headed there, forgetting the bridge I hadn't crossed in the afterglow of the one I had.

After the six miles, I returned to our room to take my first ice bath. Articles raved about reduced inflammation and less post-run pain from sinking the lower half of the body into freezing water. My legs hurt, so I was willing to try.

The Penguins explained how to make it tolerable. Instead of filling the tub and then getting in and shocking yourself nearly to death, they suggested a process similar to the desensitization I'd just done for my anxiety. I crawled into the empty tub naked and turned the water to the coldest setting I could tolerate. As the tub filled, I turned the water colder and colder, allowing my body to acclimate. Earlier, I'd filled the ice bucket and trash cans with ice and put them next to the tub. Taking care not to splash, I added handfuls of ice until the frigid water covered my waist. I shivered there, goose-bumped, but not screaming, for ten minutes. Some folks recommend more time, but that was enough for me. I hadn't yet read about wearing a sweatshirt to keep the upper body warm. Maybe I'd try that later. For now, I'd endured this rite of passage—one step closer to being a real runner.

CHAPTER 12

Tying Myself to the Planet

By April 9, a little more than a year after I'd taken up running again, the winter storms were mostly over, and leaves had begun to sprout. Cold, brisk, and cloudy, it was a fabulous day to pin on a race bib and close the Hundred Days Challenge with the Tin Man 5k. The wind whipped the sixty of us waiting for the gun. We wound along a partly paved, partly gravel trail in a metro park amid tall grasses, over bridges, and around a big pond. I cheered a friend doing the 10k where the courses crossed. Feeling much stronger than I had in the New Year's Eve "pink hoodie" race, I easily set a PR. Ed took pictures and yelled, "Go Nita!" I liked making my heart pound. Perhaps I was becoming an athlete.

***

The week after my happy Tin Man 5k, I learned that a friend had died of a heroin overdose, possibly a suicide. He and I had attended the same weekly recovery group for years. His death stunned everyone who knew him, myself included. A few days later, a friend's boss shot himself in the parking lot of a nearby police department. Both events rattled me. While mourning the losses, I worried the knives in the kitchen drawer might jump out and stab me. I asked Ed to hold me. "I need to tie myself to the planet, so I don't spin off."

Ed's mood is so stable, I'm tempted to call him "steady Eddie." In the early years of our marriage, because he loves to fix things, one day, he asked me to go to a movie with him to snap me out of the doldrums. He had previously suggested I volunteer at a soup kitchen, but I didn't have the energy for that.

We watched *When a Man Loves a Woman*, starring Meg Ryan and Andy Garcia. When recovering alcoholic Alice Green told her husband Michael, "I'm not your problem to solve," Ed turned to me, recognition in his eyes. Years of living with me helped him understand that any relief I found in movies or volunteering would be temporary. Sometimes I wouldn't be capable of those activities at all.

The night I found out my friend had died, I cried for all the people lost to addiction and depression. I explained to Ed how, when your mood rolls like a small boat at sea, the unthinkable becomes possible. I reassured him I didn't want to die. He listened, and when I finished talking, he held me until I fell asleep.

***

In the weeks before these deaths, I'd considered running the Hoover Hustle 10k to train for the Cap City Quarter, but the course crosses the Hoover Reservoir dam, which terrified me. I signed up anyway.

The night before the race, I dreamed that, halfway across the dam, trapped by fear, I froze in a swirl of clouds. Water rushed beneath me and splashed my shoes. In my dream, the middle of the dam was razor-thin. I teetered on the narrow ledge, alone, staring at the churning water flowing from the spillway. A cold wind whipped and blew me off balance. As I fell, the icy water stifled my screams. Before my head went under, I woke, gasping and sweat-covered, clenching the covers.

In the dark, hearing Ed's gentle breathing, I decided to skip the race and went back to sleep in peace.

But, in the morning, I remembered my friend who had died. My fear seemed silly in the face of his death.

I talked to Ed. "It was just a dream," he said, then realized anxiety had paralyzed me. "You can't let fear win," he added. But this would also be the first race I'd done without him.

Ed's years growing up as a blonde, blue-eyed boy in southern California had damaged his fair skin. The Friday before, he'd had a "blue light" procedure and had to stay indoors, away from light, for three days. "You can call me," he said. "Go see what happens."

This calmed me enough to get me in my car, but as I drove toward the reservoir, panic rose again. I was no match for this dam.

I turned on classical music and breathed into a paper bag as I drove. Once I parked, I reminded myself that the race started on dry ground. The dam was not for a mile. But as soon as I thought of the dam, I put my face back in the paper bag. After my breath returned to normal, I pinned the bib to my chest.

I checked my waist pack for the foil gel packets I'd brought. Gels provide electrolytes and supplement the body's glycogen stores burned on longer runs. I'd eat one if I crossed the dam. I slid the car keys in with them and stepped into the fierce wind.

Once the race began, nearly everyone passed me. To avoid looking at the dam, I focused on the runners ahead. As I moved closer, my stomach clenched, and I closed my eyes to push against it.

When I opened them, the dam was in the distance, gray concrete and surprisingly small. Even though I'd seen this dam many times during my decades in Ohio, my nightmares had distorted it into a looming structure like the Hoover Dam that separates Nevada and Arizona. I imagined it dominating the landscape, dwarfing anything nearby. I'd also forgotten that the south side was dry earth, with only a small spillway. If I panicked, I could roll down the hill. The fall might bruise me, but I wouldn't drown. The wide expanse of concrete across the dam resembled a two-lane road more than the razor's edge of my nightmares. Elated, I headed toward the middle.

On the dam, the wind picked up. My body tensed when I saw the water on my left. I sped up. My ears whistled through the headband. But, when the bicycle leading the head runner came toward me, I cheered, clapped, and jumped up and down, forgetting about the dam.

At the water stop across the dam, I celebrated by opening an energy gel. They're concentrated, so you take them with water. Ideally, I'd have tried one on a training run, but I'd not yet heard the admonition "Nothing new on race day." When I squeezed the foil packet, the gel spread over my fingers like wet glue. I licked the tasty goop and drank a cup of water. I washed my fingers in a second cup, then threw it all into the last trash can. The lemon-lime gel tasted like frosting, but it was clear, viscous, and yummy. But I'd have to figure out how not to make a mess. Thankfully, that was the only consequence.

We ran through woods and down a hilly country road marked by cones, then turned up a steep incline, back toward the dam. I locked my eyes on the man in front of me and pounded up the hill.

Over the dam I went, again, face into the wind. I turned my head to the grassy side, noticing only mild heart palpitations. I thanked the dam for not killing me and finished the race. In the post-race photo, I am radiant, with my hair standing straight up in a headband as if it had been hair-sprayed in place. My friend was dead. I would do my best to persevere.

CHAPTER 13

The Quarter

The night before the Capital City quarter marathon, Ed and I strolled through the race expo, past booth after booth of running and walking apparel. Most large races combine "packet pickup," where participants pick up their race bibs, with an "expo" of exhibitors. Ed loves expos. He'd attended many during his stint with Price Waterhouse and his decades as a Chief Financial Officer for different organizations. Here, exhibitors promoted mud runs, warrior runs, and even a run where you jumped over a pit of fire. Those races didn't interest me. Give me unicorns and rainbows. Ed may not run, but he took all the freebies and completed the contest entries anyway.

A majority of the attendees would run the half marathon, 13.1 miles. I was in awe. With my wonky ankle, I was "only" running the "quarter" marathon of 6.55 miles. The "only" was a joke. I was forty-nine years old, slightly overweight, afraid of my own shadow, and had never been athletic. Yet, here I sat with my husband, listening intently as professional athletes on "The Panel of Champions" answered questions and news folks took photos. Even though I was "only" running the quarter, when doubts arose, I reminded myself I belonged. I too knew what it was like to train and achieve. I too was an athlete.

***

On race morning, as Ed and ten thousand participants tried to park, I panicked, afraid we would miss the start. Despite Leslee's reassurance, I insisted we hop out while Ed and Leslee's husband, Kevin, parked.

My legs felt wobbly as we walked. It had only been a year since I had jogged through that isolated ravine carrying a kitchen timer with the dog at my side.

This large race had "corrals," fenced areas to which each runner was assigned based on projected finish time. Leslee tried to explain that it would take ten minutes for us to cross the start line since we were in the last corral, but I didn't believe her. So many runners in one place both thrilled and terrified me.

Next to the corrals was the longest line of porta potties I'd ever seen, with people queued four or five deep. I was used to one or two near the registration table. Leslee and I joined the line. When we came out, our corral was full, with runners in colorful spandex crowded around the corral entrance. I had no urge to join the jostling group. Leslee stood near the opening. "We'll go in once they start."

A loudspeaker blared words and music I couldn't understand. My muscles quivered with anxiety. I just wanted to start.

Although I'd already run 6 miles on my own and 6.2 miles in a race, 6.55 seemed too long. I fingered the map I'd printed, studied, and folded into my belt. But even as I reminded myself that I'd be turning off ahead of the half marathoners, so wouldn't be last overall, my stomach quaked.

Finally, as the crowd started to walk, Leslee and I merged into the corral and inched toward the start. We were at the start line before we could run. People sped past on the left and right. Their pace was infectious. "We're going too fast!" Leslee said. We both slowed.

I moved to the right, but not before a young man brushed harshly against my arm. Old, slow, and outpaced, even in the last corral. I lamented letting Leslee talk me and my bad ankle into this.

"How's it going?" Leslee asked. "I'm moving," I squeaked. We continued at our snail's pace until even walkers were passing us.

Eventually, I remembered ChiRunning. I relaxed, tilted my pelvis, and let my arms swing back and forth. I tucked my chin and lifted my chest. I made sure my foot turnover was quick and light. My mood lifted.

Near the first mile marker, some people who'd passed us earlier were lined up at the small row of porta potties beyond a water stop. I happily passed them.

The more we ran, the more confident I grew. But Leslee's breathing grew heavy, and soon I was doing all the talking. I was ready to speed up.

Before the race, Leslee and I hadn't had "the talk" where we each agreed to run our own race. I wished we had.

When Leslee said she might walk, I asked, "Do you mind if I go ahead?" Any fear I'd had of getting lost had vanished. "Go on," she said. Unconvinced, I asked again. She reassured me. "You'll probably catch me later," I said and leaned forward to increase my pace.

Cheering fans held signs ranging from "Call me! You have stamina!" to "Run like you stole something!" Live bands and DJs entertained us. A ragged man with a scruffy beard and a big coat rode a bicycle and carried a boom box blaring "Chariots of Fire" and "Eye of the Tiger." I saw him three times. He looked like one of those guys you see at the end of the freeway ramp with a cardboard sign asking for money, but he was one of our best cheerleaders. I gave him a fist pump, which he returned.

Toddlers held out their hands for high-fives. I slapped tiny hands until my own were sore.

Near the three-mile mark, a group of women wearing matching T-shirts passed by. Their shirts bore the name of a woman who'd died of a heart attack while training for the race. The local news had interviewed her daughters, and I'd sobbed when I'd seen it. As they passed, I called out to say I would keep the family in my thoughts. Our family had so many deaths in 2007 that these stories broke my heart.

As we neared the quarter marathon turnoff where the half marathoners would continue, part of me was relieved. Another part wanted to do the "whole" race. Someday, I thought. Just not today.

After the next turn, onto High Street, runners blew past me the way they had at the start. I wondered how they were getting a second wind. One breath in, one breath out with each stride, I gasped for air. At the water stop, people weren't even slowing down. They grabbed the cups and continued running. I wound up with most of the water down my front.

Then I remembered this was where the quarter marathon rejoined the half. The runners passing were the faster half marathoners. No wonder they were flying! I slowed and moved far to the right.

When I turned onto Nationwide and could see the finish line, I felt the usual burst of energy and sprinted. But the line was further away than I thought. I pulled myself back and still crossed happy.

A volunteer gave me a glass of water and a veteran hung a medal around my neck. Leslee wasn't far behind. Like me, she'd been swept up by the half marathoners. "They practically carried me to the finish!"

We asked someone to take our photos, then looked for our husbands. It was forty-five degrees. While running, Leslee and I were comfortable, but that temperature was unpleasant for spectating. The men had found a warm cafe in which to discuss politics. We'd finished sooner than I'd estimated, so they had missed our finish. Ed felt bad, but I was happy he'd found a friend to talk with about one of his passions.

At home, I hung my first real medal on the corner of a picture in my office, so I could see it every day.

CHAPTER 14

Marathoner in Training

In March, a year after I'd taken up running again, a local group brought *Runner's World* Chief Running Officer, Bart Yasso, to Columbus to speak. I'd read Bart's book, *My Life on the Run*, on our trip to Montreal the previous fall.

Marathoner in Training (MIT) advertised half or full marathon training groups. I didn't feel ready to train for a half but contacted Fleet Feet about Bart's visit. Jeff Henderson, head coach of MIT, encouraged me to attend the Saturday group run. Following Bart's talk, Ed stayed in the auditorium reading political history, while I pushed my fear aside and ran with MIT's slowest-pace running group on the Olentangy Trail. I quickly fell behind and finished just ahead of the walkers but didn't mind. On my return, Ed snapped a photo of me, Bart, and Jeff, who is six foot eleven and fondly referred to as "the Tall Guy." Bart's not short, but next to Jeff, Bart and I looked minuscule.

After my morning with MIT, every fourth person I talked to had trained with the group. People I didn't even know ran were members. I'd seen MIT signs at the Cap City Expo and runners wearing MIT shirts at the race. In May, I went to an MIT information session.

Thirty or forty people gathered at Fleet Feet by the wall of colorful socks and racks of tech gear to hear Jeff explain what to expect. I'd already signed up for some 5ks and worried about missing Saturday long runs. Jeff suggested I work them into my training plan. I told him about my wonky ankle and he recommended their doctor and physical therapists. When I told him I was slow, he mentioned the walkers. He shot down every excuse I had.

Back home, I wrote a list of pros and cons while Ed laughed. He didn't know I'd already spent an hour reading tarot cards, flipping coins, and turning the Magic 8 Ball I kept in the closet over and over. "Reply hazy. Try again later."

I wanted to run a half marathon. I needed the structure a schedule and a coach would provide. But I'm an off-the-scale introvert. Groups make me nervous and stressed. Still, running with MIT the day Bart Yasso spoke taught me that, even with a group, you're mostly alone. On the trail, people pair off to share the trail with cyclists. You only talk to three or four people. I could tolerate that.

And I didn't yet understand how deep trail conversations could be. Only later would I appreciate like-minded "in person" friends, not just internet buddies, to share my newfound love and to turn to for advice.

Plus, in running, the main personality I'd have to deal with was my own. There would be group dynamics, but, for the most part, I'd only be comparing me to me. That's why running suits me so well.

I marked Saturday, May 21, 2011, the start of the MIT season, on my calendar. I was about to become a (half) marathoner in training.

On the way to my first Saturday MIT workout, as I anxiously drove the freeway, a maroon SUV pulled behind me. When I changed lanes, it changed lanes. I pulled onto the exit ramp at State Route 161. So did it. I glanced at the young, ball-cap-clad man behind the wheel, my heart beating in my throat. I turned right. He did as well. Then I saw the line of cars in the left-turn lane by the Thomas Worthington High School driveway and laughed. My ball-cap-clad friend was also headed to MIT. He followed as I moved to the end of the line of waiting traffic.

The parking lot was nearly full of cars bearing 13.1 and 26.2 stickers. My car had a "Sorry, I've got to run...with my dog" sticker, so wasn't completely out of place, but I still felt shaky. A half was twice the greatest distance I'd ever run. I hoped these folks would show me how.

More than five hundred runners, including the young man with the ball cap, milled about in shorts, tights, T-shirts, running skirts, and racing singlets. A few had dogs on leashes. I hadn't brought Mr. Dawg because I didn't know what to expect.

I sat with some friends while Jeff introduced over fifty pace coaches, starting with a seven-minute-mile group and ending with the walkers. Each wore a bright "Coach" T-shirt and held a sign designating their group's pace.

I went to the slowest running pace group: thirteen-minute miles. Three coaches welcomed us: a gentleman slightly older than me and two much younger women. Thirty of us, ranging in size from petite to plump and age from early twenties to sixties, stood together. I felt downright old.

When a coach explained they were trained in CPR, I checked my pulse. Okay so far. As we walked toward the driveway, my mild anxiety surged into hypomania. I was going to train for a half marathon: thirteen point freaking one miles! These people were going to help.

Several returning women engaged in witty banter. I said a little too loudly, "You look like the cool kids. Can I hang with you?" One said, "I don't know if we're cool, but we're loud." Giddy, my mind zipped with positive thoughts. The summer sun sparkled. I felt witty and bright.

As we jogged toward the Olentangy Trail bike path, everyone passed me. One of the pace coaches fell back to make sure I was okay. I assured her I was but explained that I couldn't keep up. "Just do your best," she said, then went to the next person up the line. Another coach kept the pace from the front.

I had to leave early to teach a writing class, so I asked a young man with a GPS watch to let me know when we'd run half a mile. When he did, I turned around and ran back up the tree-lined trail and the driveway to the stop sign where we'd begun. Pride filled my heart.

While MIT had a lot of members, the small pace group seemed approachable. I only needed to talk to the person running beside me. Besides, I wasn't talking. I was huffing and puffing, hoping my endurance would grow. Since I'm bipolar Type II, I don't get the kind of mania where you max out your credit cards or engage in dangerous activities. Rather, I look and feel optimistic and outgoing. When I'm not hypomanic, I'm usually depressed. Being hypomanic that day made what might normally feel overwhelming seem easy. I might regret it later, but it was too late. I was in.

***

While Morgan couldn't join MIT, he did get to race. On a hot Sunday at Fred Beekman Park, after my first Saturday MIT run, Morgan and I ran the Eye 5k to benefit Pilot Dogs while Ed walked the one-mile fun walk. About thirty dogs and one hundred people, mostly college students, took part.

Since it was Morgan's first race, I worried he would trip someone or get too hot. Worrying gives me the illusion of control. I wish it burned calories, but all it burns is my stomach lining.

At the starting horn, Morgan lunged, barked, and pulled, trying to stay with the dogs and runners quickly passing by. Whatever ancient vestiges of pack behavior remained in Morgan's canine heart stirred, and he howled, "Mom, they're getting away!" I felt elderly and exhausted. I missed our quiet neighborhood where we give dogs a wide berth.

When Morgan surged again, I yelled, "No!" a word he's not used to. I gripped the leash so he wouldn't rip it from my hands. "Mommy can't run that fast," I explained. He sighed heavily. He didn't know it wasn't about winning. We needed to pace ourselves. At least, I did.

Eventually, he settled. Others on their second lap passed us on our first. We passed a woman carrying a tiny papillon. She smiled and I waved. Morgan showed no interest in the snack-sized dog. The big dogs were still getting away.

Three-quarters of the way around the second lap, the papillon, now on the ground trotting beside the woman, passed us. Morgan pulled. I tried to keep up but couldn't hold the pace. They beat us to the finish.

Ed met us with a bottle of water. Morgan greedily nosed out a smaller dog at the first water dish, so I steered him toward a second to let the smaller dog drink.

Ed had taken a picture of Morgan and me "running." As in most race photos, I look like I'm walking. My wet, cotton, lavender animal-rescue-site tank top and my cotton capris clung to my body. The Penguins had taught me "cotton kills" in winter, but I mistakenly thought cotton was cooler.

Morgan's tail wagged heartily as I carried the large bag filled with dog food samples, treats, and toys he had scored. Better swag than most people races. I was no longer the only racer.

***

Our mail carrier watched my progress as he delivered mail, house by house. Postal carrier by day and author James D. Bethel by night, he's also a runner who coached his son's high school cross-country team. If he saw Morgan and me running, he waved. One day he greeted me with, "You training for anything?" I'd become a person who, when asked, had to elaborate. I told him about MIT.

He offered advice whenever we met. If we caught him at his truck, which Morgan heard coming, he gave Morgan a biscuit, and he and I talked while he sorted mail. Since I was no longer afraid to run in public, I liked the attention. Perhaps I was becoming my oh-so-shiny mother.

We discussed his progress on the novel and my struggles with my monthly newsletter essay. A few times a year, I left a box of dog biscuits out with the mail to replenish his supply.

He saved his holiday tips to buy a treadmill. "I need to keep running in the winter." I asked if walking his route wasn't enough exercise. "It's good," he said. "But nothing beats running."

As my training miles increased, I asked about aches and pains. "If there's no blood," he began, then corrected himself. "If there's no bone showing, keep going." When I had a cold, he said, "If you're not in the ER, keep running. The fresh air is good for your lungs and the adrenaline will push the toxins right out of your body." Hard-core, this guy.

***

I skipped a Saturday MIT for Morgan's second race, the much larger Rescue Run 5k at McFerson Commons Park. This time I wore a sleeveless aqua tech shirt and black tech capris instead of cotton.

Ed, Morgan, and I walked the exhibits, snagging biscuits for Morgan and Hershey's Chocolate Kisses for Ed. We signed up for raffles, then made our way to the start. I anticipated Morgan's start-line antics and positioned us behind the walkers. I kissed Ed goodbye and hugged my friend Lisa, since she and her small dogs were walking. The gun went off. Morgan barked and pulled but had the satisfaction of passing a few walkers.

Morgan and I caught our friends Chris and Heather with their golden retriever, Murphy, when they stopped for water. Near the finish, Chris and Murphy sprinted away. Heather and I gave chase and passed them before the finish, which Ed caught on camera.

These were "real" runners. Even though I was training for a half marathon, I said I wasn't really a runner. Heather had run a full marathon, and she and Chris both ran fast. I'd run with them! In the photo, Morgan is running full-out, his front legs reaching forward across the brick street and I'm sprinting. For the instant Ed captured in the picture, I felt like a "real" runner.

***

As part of my quest to heal my ankle and manage my anxiety, I had a massage each month. MIT folks talked about the benefits, and I'd long heard it was good for relaxation, so I bought a membership at a franchise center. My first massage therapist, a young, energetic runner, stretched my muscles. He suggested soaking my ankle in Epsom salts, wrapping it at night, and keeping it elevated when possible. "It's just inflamed," he said. "Once that goes down, you can really move it." He didn't think running at my age or weight was a problem.

But he left. I hadn't gotten his full name, and they wouldn't provide it. They next paired me with a woman who'd just run her first 5k. While she didn't stretch me or suggest anything for my wonky ankle, she gave a good massage, and encouraged my running.

When she left to start her own massage center half an hour away, I asked for another male therapist, thinking he might be like the first guy. But he complained non-stop. I asked for someone different and they scheduled me with another lackluster person. Finally, the center paired me with a therapist who believed in holistic remedies, gave a great massage, and offered the kind of support I'd received from the other therapist.

When she left, I cancelled my membership.

***

Each Memorial Day during the decade we'd lived in Upper Arlington, I'd awakened to neighbors cheering the runners in the Memorial Day Five-Miler that winds through our community. One race morning, I'd squealed my car tires and sworn at volunteers when I'd found the streets blocked. Now, after I'd run a few races, traffic control made sense.

This year, I intended to thank every volunteer to make amends. The four-hundred-person road race, the oldest in central Ohio, draws a fast crowd, and the temperature is rarely below eighty degrees. I'd just run the day before, and five miles exceeded my weekly MIT training plan. Scared I'd be last, I started too fast, especially for the heat. I barely stayed ahead of the police escort.

A group of police officers in training started at the back of the pack and jogged the entire five miles. They chanted, "Left. (Pause.) Left. (Pause.) Left. Right. Left." I was glad when they passed by, as I cherished the silence of being nearly alone.

The first water stop ran out of cups. A little boy threw a handful of water at me and laughed. I cupped my hands under a jug spigot, sipped from my hands, and moved on, still thirsty.

Near the three-and-a-half-mile mark, Ed and Morgan waited on our neighbor's lawn. When Morgan saw me, he barked and twirled.

Despite my thirst, when I realized Ed was recording me running up the hill, I waved bravely. A few houses down, Colin Gawel, a local rock star and coffeehouse owner, and his family had set up a makeshift water stop. Colin's son sprayed me with a hose, and I sucked down a big cup as Colin picked up the empties.

I beat my five-mile Turkey Trot time by eight minutes. Tired, achy, spent, and sunburned, I drank water and herbal iced tea the rest of the day and worried I'd done permanent damage.

***

I'd missed two MIT Saturdays because of the weekend races and attended the Wednesday MIT run to perk me up. I was back in the habit of sleeping until noon and keeping the blinds closed all day.

Fewer than fifty people were in the parking lot on Wednesday night, and no one was from my pace group. Participants formed two groups near the stadium: the uber-trim, sinewy speed-work folks and the "casual runners." I quickly fell behind the casual runners. I didn't have a GPS watch, so I didn't know when to turn around. The run/walk group pace coach kindly joined me. I struggled to keep up and turned when she did. While I appreciated her gesture, I would have preferred to run through our neighborhood with Mr. Dawg. Part of my sadness was the memory of his pouting face when, after he smelled my running clothes, I left without him. "Unbelievable!" he'd muttered, wondering what he'd done wrong.

I pushed aside the "You don't belong" thoughts as I drove home. I hugged my husband, scratched the dog, and logged a successful workout.

Some Saturdays, when I ran with MIT, I fell behind. Other days, I kept up. It bothered me, but I showed up regardless. When I asked Duane, the pace coach closest to my age, about my slowness, he said not to worry. "No one will force you out." I'd wanted him to tell me how to keep up, but if I pushed hard, jarring my body, my ankle, knee, and hip ached. Still, I worried I wasn't working hard enough.

When I ran with Morgan, he stopped and started to pee and sniff, so I ran more slowly than on Saturdays with the group. Ed suggested

I train the dog to only pee once, but I didn't have the heart. Him sniffing for wild animals and trash was like me reading the paper. I would never keep him from this joy.

By the end of August, as the MIT distance increased, several others in our group also fell behind. Grumpy folks complained the coaches were too fast. I didn't know. My watch didn't show pace, only the time. I estimated the distance. During the week, I continued using the website maps. I might not have been running any faster with MIT. My method of keeping track might have just been inaccurate. My mind always needs something to worry about, and this filled that need. Since Duane had reassured me, I tried to stop focusing on pace and just feel grateful to complete the miles.

Besides pace, clothing, and wonky ankle problems, I had a peeing problem. Sometimes I went for a long run and didn't have to pee at all. Other times, I barely made it to the first porta potty. Remembering the joke I'd made at the Turkey Trot about Depends, I bought my first package.

I befriended another first-timer, Kelley, who had a welcoming smile and bright eyes. The miles along the Olentangy River trail flew as we laughed at my bathroom breaks, discussed books we were reading, and lamented the state of the nation. Another back-of-the-packer, Stephen, and I planned upcoming projects in the organization to which we both belong outside of MIT. Because of his intense demeanor, Stephen's humor surprised us. He and I shared the perils of running while "older" yet feeling younger than our chronological ages. Kelley, Stephen, and I forged friendships as we sweated out the tough runs and laughed on easy days.

One morning after our long run, when neither Kelley nor Stephen was there, a chatty runner named Sarah invited me to breakfast with the pace group. I asked three times if she meant it. I try to hide my paranoia, but sometimes it breaks out in public. She reassured me. I enjoyed the eggs, coffee, and lively conversation as the more experienced runners shared their adventures.

When the heat forced Saturday runs to six thirty in the morning, I griped but went anyway. That sleep-'til-noon person had found a community to help her chase her dreams.

CHAPTER 15

The Big "Five-Oh!"

The summer of 2011 brought my fiftieth birthday. Life wasn't perfect, but fifty didn't scare me. At forty-five, I'd been miserable—thirty pounds heavier, inactive, and often suicidal. Now, I'd lost weight and was keeping it off. We'd been back in Ohio for over ten years and were still happily married. I'd made peace with the deaths of so many loved ones. I felt thirty, not fifty.

I attributed this to running. My psychiatrist continued to believe running allowed me to stay on a lower dose of antidepressants. In 2000, when we'd moved back to Ohio from New Mexico, I'd been on six medications. Now I was on low doses of three. I daydreamed about quitting them altogether, hoping I'd lose twenty pounds, but I'd tried to stop three times before, with disastrous results. With each experiment, I was fine for a while. I regained my full range of emotions and lost weight. But eventually, panic and anxiety crept back, followed by a crippling lack of energy and sour mood. Anxiety and depression flipped like two sides of a well-worn coin.

To remember why I take my meds, I simply recall a day in New Mexico when I had an urge to hurl myself through our gigantic plate-glass window so strong that I ran into the yard and lay in the dirt until it passed. The following day, I buried myself in bed while fending off thoughts of driving my car the four miles from our house to the Rio Grande Gorge Bridge, a popular location for suicide. The next day, I paced the long hallway of our hillside bi-level with racing thoughts and a trembling body. That anxiety brought no weight loss, since I was also bingeing on ice cream.

Even with my wonky ankle pain, I felt content. Running hadn't cured my depression or my obsession with food. It hadn't helped me finish a book. It hadn't allowed me to quit taking meds or seeing my therapist, but I felt more peace. Instead of sleeping until noon every day, I only slept until noon on days when I didn't run. Instead of skipping bathing, I showered every day I ran. On days I didn't run, I often wrote. My emotions still rolled like the waves beneath a ship, but at least I had self-esteem on the days when I ran or wrote and didn't constantly think about food. Despite the periodic ankle pain and my periodic doubts about whether my wonky ankle would hold up to half marathon training, life had improved.

***

By my fiftieth birthday, my cushioned Brooks Adrenaline shoes had far surpassed their three-hundred-mile life span. I fixated on finding shoes to help me run without injury. Articles I read supported flatter, less cushioned shoes, like the water shoes I sometimes still ran in. Focusing on running form and strengthening your feet with minimalist shoes was the new trend, although the science was fuzzy.

I fell in love with the light, flat Merrell Pace Gloves. Like the water shoes, they had no heel and little sole, but they were an actual shoe. I carried both the Adrenalines and the Pace Gloves to the gym to test the Pace Gloves on the track, where it would show less wear in case I needed to return them. I ran in the new shoes for half a mile, then switched. I gradually increased the distance in the Merrells and stopped wearing water shoes.

Meanwhile, the swelling in my ankle varied. For weeks, it wouldn't swell at all. Then one day it would swell for no reason. In the Merrells, my ankle sometimes clicked. It never clicked in the Adrenalines. My health care practitioners thought my ankle was acclimating to flatter shoes. The change to a midfoot strike needed to be gradual. Race photos showed me still heel-striking, but had been taken near the finish, when I was sprinting. If I tried to go fast, I bent at the waist and came down hard on my heels.

The lack of flexibility in my ankle showed up as pain in my left knee. This was also intermittent. Tilting my pelvis ChiRunning style helped, but wasn't an absolute fix.

I decided the Pace Gloves were too minimal, so I tested several pairs of "in-between" shoes on the track. Eventually I settled on Brooks Ravenna, another cushioned shoe with a heel, but one which didn't make my ankle click. It was less minimal than I wanted, but flatter than the Adrenalines.

***

In July, a Newton Shoes representative taught form exercises at our local Fleet Feet store. A sale on top of my regular running-group discount convinced me to buy a pair. Newtons have a low heel but are cushioned. Even though I'd lost weight, I was still large for a runner, so cushioning was recommended. An Athena, they call a larger woman runner. The larger men they call Clydesdales.

On the track, in the Newtons, my ankle clicked, but not as much as in the Pace Gloves. Since articles claimed that rotating shoes prevented injury, I began rotating the Pace Gloves, Newtons, and Ravennas. Plus, it made me feel like a real runner.

My ankle didn't swell in July when we visited Ed's son in Carmel, Indiana. I ran the Monon Trail using the metronome at 159 beats per minute, focused on form. Half a mile in, the pain subsided. By early August, if I focused on form, my ankle didn't click. I was still rotating shoes but liked the Newtons for longer runs.

Then it turned hot. When I ran seven miles alone on Saturday, my whole body ached. I couldn't imagine running twice that far. Another day, while I waited for the mechanic to repair my car, I ran at Fred Beekman Park in Pace Gloves. My feet found every painful bump in the road.

On another August morning, even though it was cooler, running hurt. Left knee. Left ankle. Both shins. Left hip. I hobbled like an old lady. I tried to focus on form, but it was laborious and painful. My mind screamed, "This is too hard!" I kept running.

After that run, as I walked Morgan around our block, I saw a friend sitting in her car. We talked, then Morgan and I crossed the street. On the sidewalk, vanity took over. Even though I'd just finished a painful run, I took off. When the friend's car passed, I waved and smiled as if sprinting were the best thing in the world. When they were out of sight, I resumed walking and shook my head. I'm such a show-off.

As I gradually increased the distance in the Newtons, my ankle stopped clicking. Still, any time I had pain, I alternated between elation and certainty that I was permanently injuring myself. By the last week in August, my ankle only clicked in the Pace Gloves.

At MIT, Kelley and I talked our way through our group's first nine-mile run, despite my having knee and hip pain. The next day, when my three-mile run was agony, I remembered why I had quit running before. Form modifications made a difference at first, but as the miles on the schedule increased, the pain gradually came back, despite my cutting back the midweek runs from four to three miles. By August 29, my ankle was once again the size of a grapefruit. I'd been sitting for two days straight at a writing workshop. I believe this was a factor. My mind spun with possible causes, and I worried I'd once again have to abandon my beloved sport.

With my ankle still swollen on August 31, I told Ed I needed to go to a sports medicine clinic to determine if I had fractured my ankle. He gently reminded me that I already knew what was wrong. The pain was dull, not intense. I needed to increase mobility, but gently. On the days when I wasn't convinced I'd have to quit running altogether, I doubted I could complete the half marathon training.

***

I continued to seek a solution to my running pain. Over the Labor Day weekend, when Ed and I traveled to Santa Monica for my nephew's wedding, I went to the Egoscue Clinic for an assessment. I've used the Egoscue Method "e-cises" since the early 1990s to manage back pain. There are no clinics near Ohio.

The clinic looked like a cross between a yoga studio and a physical therapy center. Several men and one woman lay on the floor, each with one foot hanging off a wooden tower and the other leg bent at a ninety-degree angle across brown foam squares, in the e-cise I knew as the "supine groin stretch." I'd learned it from *The Egoscue Method of Health Through Motion*, my introduction to Egoscue.

Shoulders, hips, knees, and ankles should form level, ninety-degree angles. The head should perch with a slight curve atop the shoulders, and the arms should hang evenly, with the elbows and wrists parallel. Egoscue e-cises gently let gravity bring the body back into alignment.

Kai, the therapist, took photos of me standing against a straight line on a wall. My lower right shoulder and higher right hip created an unnatural curve. When I walked, instead of walking straight ahead, I went sideways, then acclimated, then went sideways again. Kai promised that e-cises done faithfully would restore my posture, help me run faster without injury, and improve my ankle. Even though my ankle bones were too close together, he believed that, in time (he always emphasized the time factor), e-cises would improve my running. He saw no danger in my training for a half marathon. I signed up for a series of Skype sessions.

***

That weekend, I needed nine miles. Kelley and I had run that far two weeks before, but now, alone in Santa Monica, my hands trembled as I fastened my watch. Even though Columbus, where Ed and I live, is the fifteenth largest metropolitan area in the United States, I still get nervous in big cities, afraid I will get mugged or lost. I chose a route by the ocean, hoping to see other runners—friends I hadn't yet met.

While Ed walked to Santa Monica Promenade, I ran five blocks to the pier, then along the concrete walk through Venice Beach to Marina del Rey and back. Medical marijuana stands, bodybuilders, and vendors selling T-shirts, sunglasses, and souvenirs lined the path. Music blared from bars. Danny Dreyer's voice on the ChiRunning CD kept me calm as I wound through alleys when the ocean walk gave way to sand.

As usual, my fears were for naught. Other runners, cyclists, and walkers, both tourist and local, passed. A large group of runners in "LA Leggers" shirts ran in clumps. I wanted to yell, "I'm in a group, too, training for a half!" but maintained a modicum of self-respect instead. I nodded and they nodded back. We were all real runners.

The sun kissed my skin and the air caressed my arms, legs and face. Running feeds my love of the outdoors. Nature, crisp in winter and hot in summer, soothes me. Whether it's the beach, the woods, or our suburb, changing landscapes, or even the same old route, Mother Earth heals. And, regardless of where I am, it feels like flying.

The next day, my husband and I met our friends Ed and Jennifer at Rose Bowl Park. Ed walked with the other Ed and I ran, while Jennifer walked faster than I was running. I tried to immerse myself in our surroundings and conversation, but my competitive mind reduced me to a fat, middle-aged Midwesterner. Never mind that she was taller and had longer legs. I judged myself for how hard it was to keep up.

Jennifer, a long-time writing friend from the workshops in Taos, complimented me on my running and weight loss. In my mind, I still weighed two hundred pounds. If she'd known I was so negatively comparing myself, she would have intervened. I wasn't in the mood to be dissuaded. As my mind grew louder, my ankle and knee hurt. Soon the messages roared, and I grew quiet, unable to concentrate. Jennifer asked what was wrong. I told her the additional training miles wore me out. That was also true, but it was mostly my negative thoughts. Even though I'd run a strong nine miles alone along the beach the day before, I slipped into a deep funk.

On our second lap, as she confided a troubling situation, I turned listening into meditation. I focused on the lilting sound of her voice, the sycamore, live oaks, and cottonwoods, and the people moving about. Each time my mind slid into self-criticism, I returned to the curve of a leaf, the red of a flower, or the sensations of my feet, slow as they may be, carrying me along. It took only half a lap before the darkness subsided, and I was enjoying her company and the brightness of the day. At the finish, the lovely faces of our husbands became my focus.

CHAPTER 16

My Mind Is Trying to Kill Me

Back in Ohio, summer turned to fall, and the miles increased. This Saturday, our group needed ten—my first double-digit run. As usual, I woke afraid I would fall behind and get lost. Unlike most of our runs, this route had turns. I still didn't have a GPS watch and didn't know the turnaround landmark. My friends couldn't remember either.

I fell behind and panicked at being alone. Trying to keep the group in sight, I ran through water stops and caught them when they paused to turn around. But running hard left me spent, and I still had to run that same five miles back to my car. I reminded myself that I knew my way home, but by the time I passed Antrim Lake, I was gasping again, certain it was heart failure. To calm down, I returned my focus to form: Egoscue technique of shoulders back and down. ChiRunning pelvic tilt. Chin tucked, with eyes on the horizon. My energy rose, and the form focuses kept the pain at bay. On the road leading to the high school, I summoned enough energy to run the hill to the stop sign. Several members of the pace group high-fived me on my first ten-miler. I wasn't alone after all.

***

In my continuing quest to solve my wonky ankle and prove the orthopedic surgeon wrong, I continued to see my chiropractor, who rotated and sometimes cracked my ankle and toes. And I added an osteopath to my roster of health care professionals.

In the osteopath's office, a colorful metal mobile hung from the ceiling to calm small children and anxious adults like me. As I lay on the table, he lifted my left foot, cradling my ankle in his hands. I admired the shapes and hues of the mobile and the way it caught the light as it turned. When he turned my ankle, it burned. I glared at one deep purple geometric metal curve and squeezed my eyes shut. He didn't stop until I yelled "Holy shit!" and pulled my foot away.

I wish I'd asked him to work more slowly but couldn't bear more pain. Perhaps continued treatments would have been effective. Instead, I continued going to my chiropractor, who also hurt, but much less, and continued icing and wrapping the ankle when it swelled. I also continued to run.

***

One afternoon, after lying on the floor during an Egoscue Skype session, my head spun with vertigo. Shaky and nauseous, I crawled into bed to let my stomach settle. In the days before I'd taken up running again, I would have easily fallen asleep. If I snuggled under the covers with the dog at my feet, dreamless slumber came quickly. This day, the thought came that I would feel less like a blight on the face of the earth if I ran instead. It was so odd that I sat up. The dog jumped down and looked up expectantly. I lay back, trying to push the foreign thought away. The dog sighed, jumped back on the bed and made himself comfortable. Instead of sleep, I sensed the gentle sway that happens during a run.

Reading my restlessness, Morgan hopped off and rubbed against the bed. "Let's go!" When I threw back the covers to put on running clothes, he bounced and galloped up and down the hallway. We ran. Afterward, I felt tired, but refreshed.

***

In mid-September, a month before the half marathon, Morgan and I ran the Second Annual Steps for Sarcoma 5k. This year, my sister Amy was in the hospital, and none of my family members could take part. I wanted to cancel and go sit with her, but she told me to run for Jamey. Plus, this second year marked the beginning of a streak. I'd run so many 5ks since that first race a year before, I felt like an old-timer.

Before Morgan and I left home, I dodged him as he jumped around while I pulled on running clothes. In the car, he whined, barked, and bounced until I let him out at the park. Against my better judgement, I allowed a race volunteer to put Morgan in a bright green T-shirt. He looked cute, but as he ran, I thought it interfered with his stride. After a quarter-mile, we stopped to remove it.

Those long runs had built our endurance. When we crossed the finish line, a volunteer asked my age, then gave me a medal for third female age fifty to fifty-nine. Amazed, I called Ed. He was at the humanist brunch group he'd organized and announced my award to his friends. At home, I checked the results to find I was not third, but fourth by seconds. I emailed the organizer, who contacted the woman who had earned the medal. Incredibly, she didn't want it. I kept it, but put a note on it saying "fourth place." Stopping to remove Morgan's shirt had cost me third.

***

During one midweek run, a new pain arose in my right knee. Then a right shin splint erupted but just as quickly went away. My left ankle felt like a block on the end of my leg. Plus, I had to cut the run short by a mile to be on time for a massage. That created havoc in my head, because I'd set a goal and not met it.

As the run mileage increased, I grew more tired. I wasn't fit enough to maintain the pace over longer miles. And pain reduced my pace even more. I had trouble maintaining good form and sagged even on shorter runs. Once again, I had to accept running more slowly.

Then, on an otherwise pain-free weekday, while wearing earbuds, I moved to the middle of the road to give a wide berth to a man mowing his lawn with a big rider. I didn't see or hear an approaching SUV until the huge vehicle blew past. I can usually hear through the earbuds, but not over a mower. The rush of air as the SUV whooshed by terrified me and spooked Morgan. I began to leave out one earbud. But it morphed into a weird fear of landscapers. The noise and my paranoia about strangers made me afraid to go outdoors if a lawn company was working on our street. I waited until they left before taking Morgan for a run.

As the season progressed, my pace slowed, while Kelley, my MIT buddy, got faster. On our eleven-mile run, I was determined to keep up with her. She didn't know where we were going either, but I wouldn't panic if I was lost with someone else.

Our long runs had fostered comfort. Talk turned to politics, religion, childbirth, sex, pet peeves, and our favorite topic, digestive processes. But there's amnesia after a run. We spent two and a half hours together and I only recall scant details of our conversation. I wonder if it's the same as childbirth. Perhaps the reason "what happens on the trail stays on the trail" is that we can't remember.

I kept up with Kelley to the turnaround and back to the Park of Roses and the porta potty I desperately needed. I told her to go ahead. Pain had started in my stiff left ankle, then moved into my left knee. By the end, my butt was screaming. I had to talk myself through, but I finished.

Afterward, part of me prided myself on my real runner pains. Another part was convinced I wasn't meant to run at all. "A real runner would be able to keep up." My brain spun. "Badass! Loser! Badass! Loser!" I reminded myself, "You ran eleven miles. That's farther than ever before." It had been difficult, but I was now confident I could run an additional two miles, the distance of a half marathon.

***

Kelley and my running friends knew little of my life beyond our Saturday morning runs. I'd spent the past twenty years creating accommodations that make me appear normal. I'm not ashamed of my disabilities. I simply want to get as much out of life as I can. My new friends did not know I had trouble getting out of bed, only showered after I ran, or had panic attacks.

Two weeks before the half marathon, while driving to a recovery meeting, I clutched the steering wheel with one sweaty hand while holding a paper bag over my mouth with the other, as anxiety-fueled adrenaline surges flooded my body. Unable to face the I-70/I-71 interchange near downtown Columbus, I took a detour that added twenty minutes to my drive. Knowing this might happen, I'd allowed extra time, but arrived shaken and spent. I told only Ed.

Because of my inability to focus, Ed winds up doing most of the household chores. I'm often overwhelmed just unloading the dishwasher or changing the toilet paper roll. When we travel, Ed navigates airports, ensuring we arrive at the right hotel, since I sometimes forget where we're going. And his emotional support is unparalleled. Once, when I was feeling guilty about how much of the burden he carries, I asked if he resented it. He explained that he'd been single for five years before we met and had grown accustomed to doing everything himself. He considered the few things I did around the house a bonus.

Unlike Kelley and some of my other running friends, I didn't have children to raise. Other than my love for Jamey, my biological clock never went off. After our Saturday runs, I could lie down. After a race, I faced depression, not hungry children. Mr. Dawg might want dinner, but I didn't have to cook it.

I'm also fortunate and grateful to have excellent mental health care when others don't. I take nothing for granted. This allows me to "show up" for things like running, writing workshops, and meditation retreats, when I might otherwise be in a psychiatric ward.

Running was rapidly becoming part of my mental health tool kit. When I ran, some of the anxiety, depression, and mania dropped away. Running helped me focus, calmed me, gave me a sense of accomplishment, and brought joy. It allowed me to achieve small goals. I set out to run x number of miles and did it. I put my fears aside and showed up. Some days, the only peace I found was in feeling my feet pound the pavement alongside Mr. Dawg and my running buddies. When I finished, it gave me the courage to show up at my desk to write.

***

Needing only one potty stop on the eleven-miler convinced me my Depends days were over. On a short midweek run, I didn't wear them, and, with each step, urine leaked down my black leggings. Maybe

I'd had too much coffee. Maybe it was the sips I took from my new Simple Hydration bottle. My mind screamed, "You're an old lady faking being young. You have no business running a half marathon." I was thankful it was just the dog and me and not a Saturday with MIT.

Then I spotted a neighbor trimming his shrubbery. I cringed when he saw us, hoping he wouldn't notice my wet legs. But he clapped and yelled, "Way to go! Keep it up!" Piss be damned. The dog and I turned the corner to our house and the longest walk up the drive. Once inside, I ran to the basement and dumped my nasty clothes into the washer with extra soap. We're runners, dammit! Morgan and I are runners.

**

Two weeks before the race, we "tapered" into lower mileage. Morgan and I ran a five-miler I thought would kill us. While listening to an audiobook on my phone, the pain in my left knee flared. When I run with distractions, I lose my form and the pain increases. About a mile in, it began to rain, cold and cutting. It dripped off the dog's ears onto the pavement. My mind yammered, "You'll catch pneumonia. You're ruining your body." I considered a shortcut but couldn't let my mind win. I looked down at the "angel wings" pattern on Morgan's back. If Jamey, Mom, Dad, and the others had been alive, they would have cheered. The pain wasn't that bad. The rain wasn't that cold. We sped up. I began to sweat, and the rain became refreshing. My satisfaction at finishing was sublime.

**

The following Saturday, MIT had twelve miles on the schedule. When one of our pace coaches advised us to only run eight, my mind went into battle. The hypochondriac feared overuse injuries. The perfectionist said I was lazy. I followed the more experienced runners and only ran eight.

"Only." That still cracks me up. But when the schedule says one number and I do less, my mind tells me I'm slacking. It rained again, but it was warmer and I'd worn another layer so didn't get soaked.

Maybe it was the camaraderie. Maybe it was my attitude or the fact we were "only" running eight. This different day brought a different mental state and a different experience. Because I'd been sore, I focused on form, and the run was nearly pain-free. Afterward, my left knee hurt a little and my ankle was stiff, but nothing like the pain of a few days earlier, pain I'd been certain would end my running. Over the years, therapists, meditation teachers, writers, recovering people, and coaches told me not to believe my mind, but now I drew that conclusion on my own. My mind really was trying to kill me. Running brought that truth home.

***

One thing I learned from the Egoscue Skype sessions was that my left gluteus muscle wasn't firing, a phenomenon called "dead butt syndrome." I didn't experience the kind of hip pain others talked about, but I wondered if this caused my knee pain. If my glute worked, perhaps it would take the strain off my knee.

But I wasn't doing the Egoscue exercises between Skype sessions. I may run long distances, but I'm deeply lazy. I need outside structure. Give me a running schedule or a trainer, and I'm okay. But I fail at exercises on my own, even if I experience the benefit. This happened with physical therapy and was happening again with Egoscue. I didn't give either Egoscue or physical therapy a fair shot.

My last "long" run before the half marathon was six miles with the group. There was much jittery laughter. Afraid of getting sick or injured before the race, Kelley said, "I'm going to wrap myself in bubble wrap and wear steel-toed boots until race day." I'd begun compulsively washing my hands and using my sleeve to open and close doors.

Our pace coaches told us our fears were normal. With only a week until our first half marathon, we had built-up excitement and anxiety we couldn't burn off since our scheduled runs were shorter. I'd encountered this "taper madness" before the quarter marathon. I'd be running twice as far on race day; maybe it was normal to be twice as anxious and excited.

The six-miler hurt. We ran through a hilly neighborhood to the Genoa Trail. I tried to focus on form but suffered going up the hills. Running with friends, I forgot my form in favor of lively conversation about the race expo, race day schedules, and the best place to buy throwaway clothes to peel off at the start. My entire left leg throbbed. The discomfort triggered the usual nagging doubt about finishing. When I talked myself out of that fear, my mind told me I was permanently ruining my body. I spent that weekend and the next few days sulking.

Six days before the half, Mr. Dawg and I went for what was supposed to be an easy three-miler. I was tired and hot, with no lively conversation to distract me. My back and legs throbbed. Plus, I was running in Merrell Pace Gloves, so I felt every bump on the trail and my left ankle clicked. I tried pelvic tilt, hip rotation, and keeping my shoulders down and back, but it was still painful and slow. My ribs, back, and right wrist also ached.

My mind yelled, "You cannot run 13.1 miles in this much pain!" I worried I would give up running after the half. I worried I'd die of a heart attack during or after. A guy had died five hundred feet from the finish line of the Chicago Marathon. I worried about growing older, facing aging, and a possible life without Ed and Morgan.

Even Morgan had a rough run. He mistook a landscaper firing up his diesel truck for the postman and was disappointed that he didn't get a biscuit.

I turned my attention to the scarlet leaves sparkling in the sun. I noticed the power in my legs, even though they hurt. I looked down at Mr. Dawg's happily perked-up ears. All was not lost. Any running was better than none. One mile at a time, I could do this.

Five days before the race, I began to ache all over. Exhausted, I napped instead of doing the scheduled short run. I hoped to kick whatever bug had caught me. Recurrent nightmares plagued my nap. By the next day, I had a fever, a headache, and nausea. My underarms erupted with angry welts. I went back to bed. The nausea, exhaustion, chills, and body aches blocked my obsessive thinking, and I slept for twenty-four hours. When I woke still sick and even more worried, I called the doctor.

She diagnosed a bacterial infection and inflammation of the follicles in the underarm. The day before my symptoms began, I'd shaved at the gym, then gotten in the pool, not knowing the filtration system wasn't working. My doctor wanted to prescribe antibiotics, but I didn't want to risk an antibiotic reaction right before the race. Instead, she prescribed antibiotic cream, vinegar washes, and ibuprofen. I followed her instructions and went back to bed. Each time I woke, I repeated her instructions. The fever broke during the night, giving me one day to recover before my first half marathon.

CHAPTER 17

Half Marathoner

I slept late the Saturday morning before the Sunday race and continued the antibiotic cream, ibuprofen, and vinegar washes. By afternoon, I was well enough to leave the house. I had my hair cut, then headed to the expo. My sweaty palm left a print on the handrail of the escalator, and my throat closed as I picked up my half marathon bib and official race shirt.

When I saw the line of people at the full marathon table, I pushed aside the thought that I was doing the lesser race. The hope of someday running a full stirred within me, but today I would focus on the half. A half was real.

I walked the expo aisles with members of my pace group. We shared nervous banter. Others bought T-shirts, tights, hoodies, half-zip pullovers, hats, jackets, nutrition, hydration, stickers, shoes, socks, physical therapy equipment, earbuds, books, race entries, Body Glide, wind briefs, belts, armbands, shoelaces, sports bras, sunglasses, and headbands. I bought a pair of "throwaway" gloves for one dollar. I already had a pair, but had to buy something to quell my nerves.

In one of the expo presentations, Clif Bar pace team member Star Blackford talked about breaking the race into three parts. The first third you run with your head, slower than you think possible. She warned of the adrenaline rush after the gun goes off. "It's easy to go out too fast." I remembered this from the quarter marathon. She said to run the second third with your legs. Pick up the pace and find your rhythm. The final third, she explained, you run with your heart. "If you hit the wall, summon the mental strength and emotional stamina you developed at the end of each long run. Your heart will carry you through." The poetry of this plan reminded me of lessons learned from years of writing practice and meditation. I remembered Nat speaking Katagiri's words, "Continue under all circumstances. Don't be tossed away."

I bought a pair of secondhand track pants and a fleece jacket to stay warm at the race start. Discarding perfectly good clothes is a tradition in longer races. Volunteers gather the clothes to wash and resell or give to the homeless. I spent $2.21. Now I was ready.

***

As a little girl, I liked to shine. My mother, a high school cheerleader, class valedictorian, home economics major, talented musician and singer, church choir director and soloist, cosmetics saleswoman, 4-H advisor, frequent class chaperone, and radio disc jockey, lived to shine. But two shiny people in the same house was one too many. Mom's histrionics, temper tantrums, pouting, and inconsistent shows of affection rendered me invisible. A child with a different temperament might have tried to outshine her or turned to negative forms of attention-seeking. I went mute, stayed out of the way, and became aggressively shy and hyper-vigilantly conflict-avoidant. I developed antennae four feet long that quivered nonstop.

As an adult, I was learning to shine appropriately. This impulse to be seen prompted me to post a link to the half marathon course on social media. Friends cheered me. To those friends who tire of my endless running posts, I issue a blanket apology, but I will not stop. My inner three-year-old loves applause. In every race, the spectators are clapping just for her.

***

On race morning, at the butt-crack of dawn, Kelley picked me up. As is normal before a race, I hadn't slept well so was a little grumpy. The night before, I'd compulsively checked and rechecked my race clothes, shoes, the running belt with the electrolyte gels in it and the bib attached, my underwear, my throwaway clothes, and the Simple Hydration bottle filled with a sports drink. The forecast was forty degrees and overcast at the start. Before Kelley arrived, I donned my gear.

Kelley expertly wove through traffic to the hotel garage, and we made our way to the conference room MIT had rented in a hotel near the start. Hundreds of MIT folks were stretching, sitting on the floor staring into space, standing in line for the bathrooms, eating pre-race snacks, talking, or leaning against the walls. We found our pace group, some of whom had already been there for an hour. Kelley's friend Barb, who had driven in from Dayton, joined us.

MIT also provided bag check. They would transport anything we didn't want to carry during the race to the finish. Jeff, the Tall Guy and running group leader, took a group photo, then directed us to put our bags in the truck. Kelley, Barb, and I complied, then headed for a hotel bathroom. When we returned, our pace group had left. We walked the several blocks to our corral but couldn't find them in the sea of people. The Columbus Marathon was much larger than the Cap City one I'd run five months before.

In the corral, I thought I might collapse before the race even began. Tired from lack of sleep and not recovered from folliculitis, I felt lost even though Kelley and Barb were beside me. I began to get the visual auras that precede a panic attack.

I scanned the faces of the people on the sidewalks, looking for Ed, and cupped my shivering hands over my mouth to regulate my ragged breathing. It was futile. I'd kissed him goodbye at home more than an hour and a half before. We'd planned to meet, but the crowd was huge. I turned around and around, making myself dizzy.

Then I saw his straw fedora. He was leaning against a bank building, scanning the runners. I yelled. His face lit up, and he trotted to the mesh fence and hugged me. Tears in my throat, I choked on my words as I introduced him to Barb and Kelley.

I jumped when the statehouse cannon boomed, signaling the start for the first wave of runners. There were fireworks, but we couldn't see them. I held Ed's hand until the crowd moved forward. I tugged at my throwaways but couldn't get them loose. I finally escaped the sweatpants and tried to hand them to Ed, who said, "Aren't you supposed to dump them on the ground?" That was against my instinct, but I did anyway. I kept the jacket.

Ed stayed with me as we crept toward the start. On High Street, he said, "See you at mile six," then squeezed my hand and walked away. I fought back tears as I watched his fedora move through the crowd. When I turned to Kelley and Barb, their eyes were wide. We were all alone, together.

***

As at the quarter marathon six months before, our start at the Columbus Marathon had entailed jogging, stopping, then jogging again. When we stopped, my feet felt nailed to the ground. When we moved, they lifted just fine. In this herky-jerky manner, we worked our way to the line. When I finally saw the metal starting arch, my heart pounded. With fingers poised to start our devices, Kelley, Barb, and I crossed the line together.

On the course, I relaxed. At the expo, I'd seen the motto, "Start slow, then back off." My only goal was to finish. Forget what Star said about starting out with your head. There was only my heart.

Kelley, Barb, and I told jokes and stories to pass the miles. Barb hadn't endured the long runs with Kelley and me, so we recapped our adventures. We clapped for the bands and thanked volunteers and spectators. Kelley had a knack for spotting photographers, and we waved and smiled.

What I saw most, though, was the insides of porta potties. Despite having gone to the bathroom before the race and again before the start, by mile two, I had to pee. And again at mile four, and just before six. I urged Kelley and Barb to go ahead, but they refused. They followed me from porta potty to porta potty.

The race felt like an enormous party on foot. With a band or DJ every half-mile, sometimes their songs overlapped. The haunting echo of a man playing bagpipes guided us beneath the bridge on Broad Street near Franklin Park while the strains of pop music blared from speakers on the nearby corner. A high school band played a drum cadence and their cheerleaders shook pom-poms at us on Nelson Road.

We seemed to be in Bexley forever, but this was because I was looking forward to seeing Ed and our book club friend, Linda, on the way back down Broad Street. When Linda yelled my name, I jogged onto the sidewalk, kissed and hugged Ed, hugged Linda, and sprinted back into the street to catch Kelley and Barb.

I appreciate all fans, but nothing compares to seeing someone you know during a race. The encounter with Ed and Linda lasted less than a minute, but, during those first five miles, I looked forward to seeing them. Afterward, I was ecstatic for a mile.

While I tried to focus on form, I was mostly distracted. I experienced intense pain around mile eight, but that dissipated, and soon we were in German Village, at miles nine and ten, where Columbus news anchor Andrea Cambern stood waving in front of her Schiller Park home.

Then we turned on High Street for a two-mile uphill slog to the finish. The pain returned from mile eleven to the end, but my friend Christy distracted us during miles twelve and thirteen by ringing a cowbell and cheering.

When we saw the finish, we sprinted. In the photos Kelley's father took, we look as happy as I remember. The experience confirmed my love of races. The crowds. The hoopla. The bands. Excitement and anxiety. Even the exhaustion at the end. I was ready to do it again.

At the MIT tent, Jeff, dressed in a full-body Sasquatch costume, congratulated us. What other race club has that!

I looked with awe at the full marathoners. While I couldn't imagine running another thirteen miles that day, I still had something in the tank. My dream of a full remained.

That night, MIT members clustered around tables at the back of a local grill to relive the race. I listened and shared. All the race talk might have bored Ed, the only spouse present, but I was so proud he was there.

***

On Monday, once the race was over and I'd hung the medal on the corner of the painting near my office door, I felt the letdown. The adrenaline build-up of training followed by the exciting race was exhilarating. Then...poof. The fans were gone, and the race was over. It was just me and the dog.

I was only as good as the race I was training for. The last race counted, but the high didn't last. Sure, there were bragging rights. My running the half amazed our book club folks. Some friends found it difficult to believe. Even I had surprised myself by running 13.1 miles, all on the same day. High school friends reminded me I'd always hated gym class. My family was proud, but the glow quickly faded.

This was the same blue mood I'd experienced after my first 5k. Again, I hadn't planned for the aftermath. Instead, I'd cleared my calendar, intending to rest, but couldn't focus on non-running things. The rest of life had become a support for running. I had a massage and talked to the massage therapist about the race.

I placed my medal on various surfaces to get the best shot and compiled an online album of photos from various spectators. Then I compulsively checked the comments. My inner three-year-old still wanted applause. The official race photos, which I would, of course, purchase despite the exorbitant fees, were not yet available. When they were, I spent hours scanning the unidentified photos to find images of myself, Kelley, Barb, and anyone else I recognized and added those photos to my order.

It took me a few days to remember the post-race blahs cure. Another race!

CHAPTER 18

Mortals Can Marathon

I didn't run again until the Saturday following the race. MIT was on break, but the habit of Saturday group runs was hard to break. I ran four miles with MIT folks and Mr. Dawg. I still fell behind, but wasn't alone. Even with my stiff left ankle and sensations in my left knee, I felt happy at how quickly my body recovered.

I asked Duane what schedule to run, now that the race was over. I wanted to maintain the base I'd built and run the five-mile Columbus Turkey Trot again on Thanksgiving. During training, I'd settled into the schedule. I'd still had to decide how many layers to wear and whether to listen to a podcast, since Mr. Dawg doesn't talk much, but the schedule removed the guesswork about how many miles to run. Duane suggested cutting back by ten percent. After my mind calmed down, I settled on running three days a week.

I continued obsessively rotating shoes. I'd run the half in Newtons, which are flatter than traditional shoes, but have more cushion than minimalist shoes. But I ran faster in traditional high-heeled, cushioned running shoes. In those, my feet and legs can't tell how hard they're hitting, so I endure more impact. Articles said it's not good to blunt this feedback. I was trying to reduce the amount of impact by changing my form. The traditional shoe also blunted my perception of whether that was working.

I also wanted to run more quickly, but this was relative. I'll probably always be one of the slowest runners. I don't have a traditional runner's body. Even with the weight I've lost, my size slows me down. I didn't know what to do except rotate shoes: traditional Brooks Ravenna, "in-between" Newtons, and minimal Merrell Pace Gloves. Part of me wanted to run in the Ravennas all the time, hoping I'd be faster, but my research said flatter shoes might prevent injury. There was no hard science on this, but I hoped the flatter shoes were easier on my body.

***

Ten days after the half, thirty members of our pace group gathered in race shirts and medals around a long row of tables to regale each other with race stories. Most had run the Columbus Half, and many were also first-timers. I sat across from Kelley. Between bites of food, she teased me about my bathroom stops and I teased her about her bad jokes.

When we traded seats to mingle, I began to chat with Sarah, a woman I'd seen, but didn't know well. During our conversation, I noticed that her Columbus medal was blue, while mine was orange. I squinted at "Marathon Finisher," then sputtered, "You—ran the full?"

She smiled, held up her medal, and said, "Yes, I did."

I had no reason to doubt her ability to run twenty-six point two miles. Several coaches had run fulls, but Sarah wasn't a coach. She was one of us. Her shape was more like mine than what I thought of as a traditional marathoner's. I hadn't paid attention to the "fulls," who didn't turn around where we half marathoners had. I'd thought of them as a different breed. But here she was, a full marathoner, dining with us mere mortals.

I peppered her with questions. What made her decide to do the full? How many other races had she done? What did she think about during the long miles? What was the second half of the course like? When did she know she was going to finish? I didn't ask what I really wanted to know, "Did your mind try to kill you?" Not everyone has that problem.

Sarah answered patiently, happy to relive the day. Nothing she said surprised or scared me. Nothing made her seem all that different from me, except that she had trained twice as hard and run twice as far. Perhaps it was her personality or her cheerful mood that day that made her decide not to scare a newcomer, but she made it sound doable.

I remembered my dream of earning that 26.2 sticker. Sarah was proof that a mere mortal could run twenty-six point freaking two miles. She had the medal and had told me the story. I wondered if I could do it too.

***

A few days after the post-race celebration, Kelley joined me for a ChiRunning refresher. We ran laps around a school track, the soft surface easy on my joints. Doug Dapo put us through some drills and I admired his beautiful, floating stride. My stride felt clunky and awkward, but I knew I'd come a long way from my early days.

Doug gave us pointers and plugged his marathon training program. "We'll have a different form focus every week." Instead of taking his program, I bought the new Chi Marathon book. Fully in love with my running group, I wanted to do my long runs with them. I hoped reading the book would enable me to use ChiRunning techniques more effectively while staying with my group.

Seeing Doug reminded me about a full marathon. I wanted to run several more halfs before trying a full. Maybe next year. For now, I'd continue ChiRunning, hope to run injury-free, and see how it went.

***

Back in August 1996, the day after I'd returned home from my first writing workshop with Natalie Goldberg and a year before we moved to Taos, I'd headed to Stauf's Coffee Roasters, where I often wrote. At a window table, two women wrote in spiral notebooks, then read aloud to each other. Beneath their table sat a well-worn copy of Natalie's best-selling book, *Writing Down the Bones*. I'd never seen these women before, despite my frequent trips to Stauf's, and I was starving for someone with whom to share my New Mexico experience. Wendy Drake was one of these women. Wendy, her long-time friend, Kristin, and I wrote together once a week until 1997, when Ed and I moved to Taos.

A few years later, when Ed and I returned to Columbus, Wendy and I picked up writing practice while she finished her MBA. Wendy had started running that fall and lamented that I'd stopped running before she and I met. I responded with my typical, "It's so hard on your body." Eventually Wendy moved to Boulder and discovered trail running and ultramarathons. When she visited Ohio, we met to write. She would tell me her latest running adventure. I'd nod wistfully and tell her about my walks around the block. Once she showed up with her foot in an air cast. She craves adventure and continually challenges herself.

Two weeks after the half marathon, Wendy visited Ohio. For the first time, we not only wrote together, we also ran. On our four-mile run along the Scioto River by Griggs Reservoir, I envied her Garmin 305, a brick of a thing that kept pace, mileage, and heart rate. A few times, she looked at it and said, "This is supposed to be an easy run. Let's slow down." I'd been afraid I wouldn't be able to stay with her. We talked about relationships, training, writing groups, and writing partners. When I confided my secret desire to run a full marathon, she didn't scoff. It was cloudy and could have been cooler. The river was brown and could have been brighter. Neither the ducks nor any of the handsome water-skiers were on the water, but it was perfect. My worlds collided in the best possible way.

In November and December, with MIT off for the season, I raced. Those long, slow, half marathon training miles had built muscles that translated into faster times at shorter distances. It was also a time for fun. The holidays brought back sharp memories of my lost loved ones, but races transformed a difficult time of year into multiple celebrations.

I PR'd (set a personal record) at the Columbus International Program 5k and would have PR'd the Rotary Honors Veterans 5k if I hadn't started out by trying to get my friends to name all the characters in the bad novel I was writing. I may have PR'd the Jingle Bell 5k, but the timing chip wasn't working and the recorded pace was half my usual. They thought I'd won my age group. I corrected them.

At the Columbus Turkey Trot Five-Miler, I didn't try to PR. Instead, Kelley and I chatted, reliving our first half. Neither of us could believe it had only been a month.

Then I used a three-mile run to qualify for the Lousy Medal Virtual 5k. I paid a fee, sent them my time, and they sent me a medal. I hadn't known such things existed.

Fleet Feet hosted "Hug a Runner Day." We ran the trails at Highbanks Metro Park, then had potluck snacks and hot drinks while a fire roared in the shelter house fireplace. We runners have several holidays. The first Wednesday in June is "National Running Day" and November 20 is "Globally Organized Hug a Runner Day." We'll use any excuse to celebrate.

For the Ugly Holiday Sweater Run, I wore a decades-old sweatshirt Mom had made during one of her numerous manic crafting sprees. Red-and-green plaid teddy bears with googly eyes adorned the front, and she had trimmed the edges with glitter glue. I smiled as I pulled it over my head, remembering her bent over the scrap-strewn kitchen table. I was ready to let my inner three-year-old shine. In daily life, I dress to avoid attention. It's a paranoid, introvert thing. But here, in my holiday outfit, I belonged. My women friends sported boas, tinsel, and velvet. The men wore Santa suits, holiday underwear, or women's holiday sweaters dripping with garland and glitter. The crazier, the better. Everyone took photos with Santa to post on social media.

At the Columbus International Program 5k, folks wore the garb of their home countries. A young girl dressed as Queen Elizabeth won the costume contest. I hadn't dressed up for that, since my heritage is so diverse. My father's family is mostly German, but my mother's family is so many other nationalities, I wouldn't know where to start. My "Rotary Honors Veterans" headband from a 5k drew the attention of a veteran and he thanked me for supporting that charity.

At the Jingle Bell Run 5k, I wore a pair of stuffed reindeer antlers with small bells on them, and the oversized holiday sweatshirt from the Snowflake Run. Runners wore all kinds of hats and outfits, including one runner in a full bunny costume.

A headband with "Happy New Year" in sparkling letters and tinsel suited me for the New Year's Day First on the First 5k. It matched my blue polar-fleece headband and drew compliments. That little girl inside me glowed.

***

I continued to read books about running. Our book club read
Unbroken, the story of Louis Zamperini, who'd been an Olympic
hopeful before World War II and became a prisoner of war. Since
Born to Run had been a hit with them the previous year, Ed and I sold
Unbroken to the group, promising it didn't have as much to do with
running as with World War II. I'd never be an Olympic hopeful like
Zamperini, but I related to the sweat, drive, and freedom that comes
from putting large stretches of road under my feet. I was also reading
Marathoning for Mortals by John "The Penguin" Bingham. A steady
stream of running books kept me motivated.

***

In November and December, even as I ran faster, set new PRs, and
had fun, my ankle and knee continued to hurt. Focusing on form
helped. When I hurt, I relaxed my lower legs, lifted and peeled my
feet from the pavement, rotated my pelvis, and leaned from the
ankles, not the waist. I bent my knees and kept my legs loose to let my
abdominals and hip flexors do the work. I kept my shoulders back
and down. I ran from my belly and let my head sit on my neck more
naturally than my normal head-jutting-forward slouch.

During November, I spent even more time sitting at a computer
than usual because I'd taken a writing challenge. I hadn't yet read
that sitting is killing us, but instinctively I knew a daily run didn't
overcome sitting all day, and it might contribute to the pain.

I still feared permanently injuring myself and sometimes had trouble
starting, but I rarely felt blue after a run, only before or during the
first mile. Especially once I crossed the halfway mark, my emotions
stabilized, making the pain seem worthwhile. Some friends thought I
was crazy not to see a doctor, but I kept working on form. When I did
it right, the pain stopped.

Still, on some days, my compulsion to lose weight drove me to run
fast at the expense of good form. My jeans were tight, even though
the scale stayed the same. Running made me more critical of my
shape and size because I compared myself to other runners. But I also

felt more athletic. If I concentrated on strength, my weight concerns disappeared. My obsession with food and weight hadn't vanished, but it wasn't killing me the way it had been when I'd been so thin in my early thirties. I focused on form and gratitude to be running at all.

***

I envied my friends' GPS watches. They didn't have to guess how far we'd gone, where the turnaround was, or their pace. In midstride, a runner would look at the giant black-and-orange brick on his wrist and say, "We're too fast." Another would look at her sleek green disk and disagree. I even envied those who waved a wrist in the air, saying, "Still no satellite." I could have used a phone app but was afraid my phone would die before the end of a run.

Some of my hesitancy around buying a GPS watch was due to the endless options. I wondered about a heart rate monitor. At my age, a history of heart disease on my mother's side should concern me, but I didn't understand how the watches worked. Pride kept me from asking and fear kept me from researching. Price was another problem. I hated the thought of spending hundreds of dollars on a GPS watch I might not use any more than my Timex. Plus, I'm not an early adopter. I still use a paper datebook.

But if you hang out in a barber shop long enough, eventually you're gonna get a haircut. When a member of my pace group posted a sale link on Facebook, I celebrated Winter Solstice with a Garmin 405.

I made the mistake of comparing the distances on my new watch to those of the online GPS maps or the watches of my fellow runners. My watch recorded shorter mileage than either. "We're not using Nita's watch" became the joke. We counted whoever's watch had the longest distance.

Garmin made suggestions, which I tried in vain and yelled in my running log, "Garmin says I only went X miles. Screw Garmin!" A more assertive person might have sent the watch back, but each time I thought about shipping it off with a demanding letter, there was the next race, and I didn't want to run without it. Eventually, the warranty expired. Later I would learn that race distances are based on tangents, and that even arm swing can make a difference. GPS is not exact.

The real question about owning a GPS watch was whether it made me a real runner. Tracking pace and mileage gave me geeky credibility. With my compulsive mental disorders and my love of technology, I was just as happy at the back of the pack with my hundredth-of-a-second PR as any faster runner. I recorded these details in the online app. I studied pace and watched for trends in how shoe rotation impacted speed and function. Still, I will never appreciate or use most of the functions of any Garmin watch. My using it is akin to shooting squirrels with an armored tank.

CHAPTER 19

Sophomore Slump

At the end of 2011, I signed up for both seasons of 2012 MIT, which scored me the "coveted" MIT jacket. I chose the highlighter yellow, but later, at the post-season sale, a rose jacket was on close-out, so I bought it too. "More" is always better.

Kickoff morning, as our group pounded down the Olentangy Trail in the morning light, I missed Kelley, who had gone away for Christmas. Stephen was running with our pace group now, so I ran with him. My left knee made its presence known, but I ran strong and steady. I thought of myself as a sophomore: no longer a freshman, but not an old-timer.

Several pace group members were training for full marathons. Since I'd met Sarah, the marathoner, at the post-season party, their presence no longer shocked me. I ran two miles with the halfs, then another half-mile with the fulls. They ran slightly slower, so I kept up, even though they were all younger. I wanted to be among them. Not yet, I told myself. I needed to train for the "whole" Capital City Half Marathon. I'd run the quarter but wanted to run the main race.

***

With winter upon us, I needed more layers. One rainy run, Mr. Dawg peed in every wet pile of leaves and the hood to my jacket kept falling in my face. It took a few runs to figure out what to wear and how to keep Mr. Dawg from turning a forty-five-minute run into two hours. On these rainy, cold runs, my mind said, "You're crazy. Go home," but the second half was great. I added fuchsia gloves with mitten flaps and a fuchsia thermal hoodie to my wardrobe, replacing the cotton hoodie and gloves. Running in this weather proved my determination. My ultrarunner friend Wendy said I was working on my "badass merit badge."

On the third of January, it was twenty-three degrees with a wind chill of nine! I wore a long-sleeved tech shirt, a short-sleeved tech shirt, the hoodie, long johns, long pants, a fleece headband, a fleece neck gaiter, and the gloves. My fingers and arms warmed up after the first mile. Only my nose stayed cold most of the way. One more point toward my badass merit badge.

One stunning Saturday morning, the group ran through falling snow. The runners in highlighter-colored jackets shone against the stark white. It was nineteen degrees with a wind chill of six. Antrim Lake was steaming. We needed to remember this morning come July, when we would be complaining about the heat. Richard posted, "This is a character-building experience."

But overall, that winter, my first with MIT, we had the warmest season in decades, with little snow. After that snowfall, we only had flurries and rain, but no ice. I quit the gym, since I wasn't going.

***

But, as our second MIT season moved through January, I felt insecure in the group. Kelley was pregnant and afraid of falling, so she didn't join. I tried to strike up a conversation with a few people but couldn't talk while running their pace. So I continued to run with the full marathoners, since they ran more slowly. I turned around before they finished, but the miles and time on our feet drew us closer. I looked forward to seeing them and, although this meant running the second half alone, I didn't mind. An extra mile with them built stamina.

Despite the unseasonably warm weather that made running more pleasant, January, February, and early March were agonizing because my writing wasn't going well.

It had been ten years since Ed and I moved back to Ohio from New Mexico. For the first five years, I'd flown back to Taos four times a year to continue assisting Natalie and did writing practice on my own. Eventually, I began to write about my dad.

In 1995, six months after my near-suicide, my former-track-star father
was diagnosed with terminal cancer. When I was growing up, he
had worked long hours as an engineer with the telephone company.
When he did come home, he escaped to the barn to feed the cattle
or tend the endless array of farm equipment in need of repair. In the
house, he chain-smoked and drank Budweiser out of long-necked
bottles while glued to *Mannix*, *Kojak*, and *Hill Street Blues*, or read
one of the mystery books he kept stacked on the end table, next to
the overflowing ashtray. He seemed a stranger until, for his last nine
months of life, he and I played golf on goat-pasture courses in central
Ohio. We talked about everything from how to keep a groundhog
from stealing your golf ball to what he wanted done with his remains.
When he was too ill to play golf, he and Mom moved in with Ed
and me. By the time he died in January 1996, our relationship felt
resolved. I had no regrets.

In 2005, during National Novel Writing Month, a writing challenge
in which you attempt to write 50,000 words during the month of
November, I wrote the first draft of a memoir about his final year.. I
revised the first draft during a year-long online workshop. In 2006,
still not satisfied with the book, I took it to Goddard College and
worked on it as my thesis to earn my MFA.

Then came 2007 and the deaths: Jamey, Ed's friend, Ed's father,
Jamey's cat, Jamey's father, Mom's former boyfriend, Mom's best
friend and then, in the final blow, Mom. I clung to the Goddard
College structure, numbing out by delivering forty pages to my
advisor every three weeks. "Don't be tossed away," Nat had said.
Recovery friends told me not to give up before the miracle happened.
Meditation friends reminded me to stay in the moment. I graduated
in 2008 and began collecting rejection slips from agents.

After two more years and thirty-seven rejection letters, I hired
a developmental editor. She returned the book with over three
hundred questions. Nine months after I'd taken up running, I was
still drowning in those.

***

To add to my misery during these winter months, numerous acquaintances died. Their funerals triggered recurring nightmares about losing so many family members. The pressure valve opened, and suicidal thoughts floated through my mind like clouds. Running became an escape from mental anguish and self-deprecation. On a run, when unpleasant or dangerous thoughts arose, I refocused on my breath and body sensations. I kept my pelvis tilted and my eyes on the horizon. I listened to the chirp of my clip-on metronome and kept my feet turning in time. Again, and again, I caught myself saying, "You're not a writer. Give up." On terrible days, the surgeon's words, "She's not going to survive this" morphed into "You're not going to survive this." When the thoughts arose, I gently brought myself back to my breath and body. Left foot. Right foot. Left foot. Right. If I focused on body sensations, the negative narrative stayed at bay.

The resilience and stability I'd learned from writing practice also fed my running. When it came time to show up for training runs, especially the long ones, I drew on what I'd learned. In writing practice, you set the timer and move the pen. In running, you choose a route and move your feet. This wasn't new. I'd done it before. I put on my shoes and ran.

***

About this time, I discovered a podcast which offered a much-needed dose of levity. "*Three Non Joggers*: Two runners and a mailman in a basement in Portland discussing all the issues no one finds important." While the Three Non Joggers talked about running, they also told middle-school-quality poop jokes and didn't take themselves or anything too seriously. It was difficult to berate myself or stay glum while listening.

I also started to cheer myself in my running logs. I've kept diaries of various types since my teens. Discovering "writing practice" in my thirties legitimized my obsessive need to record my life. I've filled shelves with spiral notebooks recording thoughts and daily activities. Since I primarily write nonfiction, these records serve as fodder, but they also create a false sense of security. I'm not worried about forgetting so much as wanting to relive every detail. In recording it, I live it twice. If I reread it, I relive it a third time. I don't forget the past. I write it all down.

Sparse comments in my logs became writing practice. Most runners log what works and what doesn't so they can repeat successful strategies. My entries included pace, what I wore, shoe mileage, weather, form focus, and pain. I also included any dogs or people I saw and sensory details. I ended each log with "Go, Nita!" or "Way to go!" as if I were a benevolent coach.

On one run, I heard someone yelling. A few houses away, I saw an older woman standing between a garage door and the front of a car parked in the drive. She didn't look trapped, but periodically she hollered. As Morgan and I approached, a middle-aged woman, two teenage girls, and a small brown dog ran out the front door toward the older woman. They tried to get her to go inside, but she refused. Finally, the middle-aged woman backed up the car. It appeared the older woman believed she was trapped, and the others played along. Once she was "free," everyone except the little dog went inside.

When the little dog saw Morgan, he raced toward us, barking and nipping at our heels. I yelled and a teen came back out and called the dog. It ignored her. I backed away, but Morgan stood his ground, fur fluffed. The little dog lunged at him and Morgan gave a fierce, guttural bark which sent the little dog scurrying back into the yard. "Sorry!" the teenager yelled. I pulled Morgan away and continued down the street. I wrote all of that in my log.

On days when I listened to a podcast, I zoned out, had little to log, and wound up in pain from not focusing on form. The podcast distracted me, so the miles flew, but I missed the birds, the wind, and smell of trees. My body paid the price.

***

This season with MIT, I'd chosen to run the "experienced" half marathon schedule. The beginner schedule dropped us back from twenty miles each week to ten. I wanted to maintain my fitness base.

I was afraid to gain weight, but, more importantly, the dream of a 26.2 sticker continued to float in the back of my mind.

The experienced plan included more midweek miles, while the weekend runs stayed the same. As a result, I grew tired earlier in the season. On one of the long runs, I mentioned doing the "experienced" plan. Julie, a more experienced runner training for her first full, recommended I not try the experienced plan until I'd done four or five halfs. I dropped a day from the training plan but kept running the longer midweek miles.

My knee and ankle still hurt, but the pain went away if I focused on form. I also chanted, "Hello, pain. Come, run with me," a mantra I'd read in the *Non-Runners Marathon Trainer*. Still, every log mentioned aches. On the positive side, my ankle no longer clicked, even in the most minimalist shoes, and my ankle rarely swelled. I attributed some of the pain to the amount of time I spent sitting. I iced and used Traumeel pain cream and occasional ibuprofen. When the tiredness lingered, I scaled back.

***

In mid-February, Ed and I flew west. We spent a few days in Carmel, California, visiting Ed's one-hundred-year-old aunt. Then we flew to Washington State to spend a night in Port Townsend, where I'd gone to graduate school, and a few days in Seattle, where Ed's older son lived. I agonized over running in these places, afraid I'd get lost. Even printing tiny maps to carry didn't fix the fear.

Running in Carmel, I remained tense until I saw Carmel Bay. The day was sunny and windy and the air smelled of salt. People walked and dogs romped in the sand as I traversed the path above. Each windblown cypress was a sculpture. The vivid spring green of Pebble Beach in the distance promised that spring would eventually come to Ohio. I returned to Ed's aunt's house happy, and ate one of the chewy chocolate chip cookies she baked for us. I might have had two.

In Port Townsend, Ed and I came upon three of my MFA professors at a restaurant. With the tightly-scheduled residency in full swing, the professors had little time to spare, but they took a few moments to ask about my writing before returning to their classes. Seeing them reminded me of how they and the college staff had accommodated my disability and the hard work I'd done to earn my degree.

Ed stayed at the cafe and read Sharon Salzburg's book about Buddhist loving-kindness while I ran three miles. Despite the familiarity of Admiralty Inlet, my insides quivered when I began. A mile into the run, I had to go to the bathroom. I stopped at a convenience store to use theirs and apologized that I wasn't carrying any money. The owner said, "We're here for the people." That calmed me a little, but I didn't enjoy the run until the turnaround. On my way back, in pelting rain, I happily wove through the shipping yard, past enormous wooden boats undergoing repair. As usual, the closer to my destination I got, the less I wanted to be done.

Ed's son, Ken, lived near South Lake Union in Seattle. Despite a good sense of direction, a map, people to ask, and my cell phone, I stood outside the hotel for a minute, talking myself into going. Ed waited at a coffeehouse near the lake reading *The Moral Landscape* by Sam Harris. Yachts docked by the water bore prices in the hundreds of thousands. An industrial area with huge metal ships scared me, but I followed Cheshiahud loop and wound up near the houseboats where *Sleepless in Seattle* was filmed. The footpath led onto a narrow, wooden pedestrian bridge alongside and slightly lower than a road bridge. Halfway across, I made the mistake of looking beneath the road bridge to see dark, stagnant water and rusted metal trusses. I raced to the other end, pushing out of my mind the fact that I'd have to cross it on the way back. In the distance, there came a faint roar. I turned a corner and saw the enormous expanse of I-5 towering ahead. On another day, I might have willed myself to run beneath it, but I'd already pushed my limits. I sprinted away with creepy-crawlies in my spine.

On the way back, the sun poked out of the clouds, revealing the Space Needle. I took photos and enjoyed the scenery. As I stepped onto the pedestrian bridge again, a man and woman already on the bridge greeted me. The sound of their feet on the wooden slats helped me not look beneath the road bridge again, but I still imagined trolls in the darkness. Around the next corner, the big ships still looked creepy and I sped past those too. My breathing only returned to normal once I saw the houseboats and yachts. At the coffeehouse, Ed had a latte waiting.

***

Back home in Ohio, the midweek runs during the end of February and beginning of March were difficult. That time is still usually deep winter in central Ohio, but it turned warm. One day, when the temperature hit seventy, I overdressed for a six-mile run. Within a block, I was soaked. I pushed up my sleeves and pushed down my socks but was still steaming. Other runners passed me wearing tanks. Plus, my knee hurt. My horoscope that week said I would learn from the darkness. Well, this appeared to be an abyss. At three miles, I thought I could go no further. At four, I alternated running and walking. My legs were like lead. I had cramps and no energy. Despite trying to focus on form, I was bent over at the waist, looking down at the ground, most of the time. I forgot why I run and wanted to quit. Usually that last mile is bliss and I run home tired but happy. That night, all I wanted to do was go to bed.

On a three-mile run, I once again forgot to wear a pad and once again peed my pants. I walked and cursed the last mile, hoping not to flood my shoes. At home, I stripped and put every stitch of clothing in the washer. I climbed in the shower, soaped myself, and cried.

One windy day, as I staggered down the street, I considered turning back. But by this time, I'd signed up for the Cap City Half Marathon, my next goal. Having a training plan made it easier to just run, not think. Despite the agony, I looked at the schedule and ran the miles.

I usually enjoyed Saturday runs with the group, but one Saturday, anxiety strangled my breath. Panicked, I tried to hide it. Julie, with her social-worker insight, recognized it immediately. "Can you feel your feet?" she asked. She'd taken to calling me by both my first and last name. In soothing tones, she repeated, "Feel your feet, Nita Sweeney. Feel your feet." The unpleasant sensations subsided, and the miles passed quickly. We talked about our families, volunteer activities, and jobs. We said it's too cold in the winter, too hot in the summer, and, on rare days, proclaimed the weather just right. We talked about whether we were running too few miles or too many, too fast or too slowly. We talked about new gear and worn-out gear we couldn't let go of because the manufacturer redesigned the model. We talked about Ohio State basketball and lamented our March Madness brackets. We talked about diets and then about what to eat after the run.

When spring hit, my running logs grew slightly more cheerful. The weather wasn't much different, but winter was almost over. On windy days, maple whirligigs showered me as I ran under sunny skies past trees lush with dogwood, redbud, and cherry blossoms. I let go of the experienced half marathon training plan and pushed thoughts of a full marathon away, choosing to enjoy the shorter mileage of the beginner half marathon plan. I still felt blue when I didn't run, but the suicidal thoughts had passed.

***

In mid-March, a representative from Newton Running videotaped us at Fleet Feet. Despite my ChiRunning practice and form focus, I was still heel-striking. I wanted to scream. He said to slow down. The key was foot turnover, he said.

I dug out my metronome but didn't know what to do differently. I countered blasts of negative self-talk with cheerleader talk and hauled myself out of the mental hole I'd dug. Maybe I'd be able to run longer distances if I weren't heel-striking and over-striding. "Think marathons," I told myself. That helped.

***

At the end of March, Ed and I traveled to DC so Ed could attend a conference and I could run the city. I spent a nervous evening plotting my route on a tourist map and reminding myself that I'd already run in other cities. After breakfast with Ed at DuPont Circle, I ran to the White House. Finding it gave me some confidence. I asked a stranger to take my photo, then ran the monuments.

I would never have attempted this adventure if I weren't running. Seeing the town on foot at my pace and moving quickly between locations, despite the other tourists, suited me. I'm not patriotic, but cherry trees fragrant with blossoms, the hum of this great city, and its architectural feats awed me like a grade school kid. Frequent stops turned my ten-mile run into four hours, but I did not mind.

Ed called mid-run, and I stopped to stretch on a bench near the Supreme Court building while he told me about a conference speaker he'd enjoyed. I told him about the reflecting pool. Two years before, I'd have stayed in the hotel, afraid to go out, or too exhausted by self-deprecation about my inability to finish a writing project to do anything except sleep.

On my tour, I practiced running meditation by remembering my form. A few times, I swung my arms in the swan-dive method the Newton Running clinic leader had suggested and focused on upright posture. I looked at the horizon, not the ground. My image in the plate-glass store window showed me landing midfoot. I hoped I was progressing.

On the drive home from DC, we spent the night at a bed-and-breakfast near Morgantown, West Virginia. The next morning, we found the Blue Moose Cafe for Ed to read more Sam Harris while I ran. Coal trucks ground their brakes to stop at the bottom of a steep hill by the intersection where I crossed the multi-lane street. The Caperton Trail ran along the Monongahela River above me.

I scrambled in gravel up a weedy hill, past litter and pieces of clothing, to the trail. "This is where they drag people to kill them," I thought. I ran north, but the steep, brambly bank to the parking lot on one side and the river on the other spooked me. It was right in town, but people get murdered right in town. I turned around. That looked more inviting, except for another bridge. I almost turned back, but knew I'd feel like a failure if I did. I continued, then crossed yet another scary suspension bridge with rusty beams and continued on to a small dam. Just before a terrifying gravel pit, the two-mile indicator went off, so I turned to retrace my path. In the cafe restroom, I took a quick sponge bath, then Ed and I headed home.

***

On the last Saturday in March, I participated in a "virtual race," the FAB run. I'd printed a bib on which I wrote, "Micah True." True, also known as Caballo Blanco, was a runner featured prominently in the book *Born to Run*. A week before, he'd gone missing during a twelve-mile run. His running was legend and the fact that he was now missing resonated with my fear of getting lost. On our MIT ten-mile run, I ran the first five with the full marathoners and five back alone, thinking of Caballo.

That evening, while having a hot flash, I went outside to cool off and admire the dogwoods in our yard. As I stepped into the grass, a sharp pain shot into the bottom of my foot. A rusty roofing tack had pierced the thin sole of my shoe, leaving a small puncture wound. I was immediately certain it would become infected and the entire foot would need to be amputated. Ed talked me out of that but asked, "When was your last tetanus shot?" I swallowed hard.

Enormously needle-phobic, I hadn't had one since I was twelve. The urgent care centers were closed, but the nurse on the help line told Ed it could wait until morning. I might have been calmer if we'd gone right away. I researched the symptoms of lockjaw.

The next morning, I tested my foot. It didn't hurt to put weight on it, so I ran the High Five Running Foolish 5k wearing the Caballo bib. The course was a loop. Participants divided into two groups. Each group began on opposite ends of a parking lot and ran toward each other, collecting high-fives. Then one group went left and the other right around the course and high-fived when we met. We also high-fived random strangers. Blue skies and cool temperatures made it perfect for silly, high-fiving fun. I pushed periodic Caballo and tetanus shot thoughts away as I ran with a new friend who talked excitedly about having just received her nursing degree. I did not mention my tetanus shot. We finished in front of only a few walkers.

I'd brought Morgan and learned how difficult it is to high-five people with him on leash. Mr. Dawg obediently runs on my left side, and we did fine so long as the recipient of the high-five was on my right. When people approached my left, however, I had to switch hands and properly time the raising of my arm for the high-five. I tripped several times while the unfazed dog endured the high-five silliness with his usual detached accommodation.

As I drove home, hands sweating on the steering wheel, thoughts of Caballo and the shot returned. No more stalling. At the Upper Arlington Urgent Care, the kind nurse let me crawl into Ed's lap. I buried my face in his chest and held my breath. After the tiniest pinch, she said, "All done." Foolishness and crazy relief swept through me as decades of bottled-up phobia vanished. I was so relieved not to have had a panic attack. I attribute this change to the overall calm I get from running.

A few days later, they found Caballo's body next to a stream in the Gila Wilderness in New Mexico. They carried him out on a white horse. Caballo Blanco means "white horse" in Spanish. An autopsy would reveal a heart deformity which some experts believe resulted from his extreme running. Although he regularly ran fifty to one hundred miles and seemed invincible, he was dead. In photos, his smile radiates compassion. I felt sad for all who loved him and silly for being such a baby about a tetanus shot when this man who had done so much for the Tarahumara Indians had died. I hoped his loved ones would find comfort that he died doing the thing he loved most but knew from my own grief that this knowledge wouldn't be enough.

***

Into April, the days grew warmer. I still had knee pain, but it continued to respond when I focused on form. I might have to accept pain as a constant companion. It seemed a worthy trade-off.

During one April run on the Genoa Trail in Westerville, Sara, our pace coach, whose mother had died while training for Cap City Half Marathon the year before, muttered "I hate this trail!" After the run, someone explained that Sara's mother had died nearby, and it was the anniversary of her death. I gave Sara a hug and told her I would continue to keep her family in my thoughts.

During the next few runs, I felt short of breath and lightheaded, definitely an undiagnosed heart condition. Eventually the symptoms passed and I chalked it up to hypochondria.

In the middle of our last long Saturday run, I asked Julie and Sue, the women I'd run with most of the season, if they thought I could run a full marathon at my age. Had I said that out loud? Julie thought a minute, then replied, "Train and see what happens." She understood my nervousness. They were both training for their first full, following the training plan, putting in long miles, and impressing the hell out of me and others. Our upcoming races, my second half and their first fulls, were three weeks away. Maybe in a few years, I thought. The full was a distant dream but saying it out loud brought it closer.

CHAPTER 20

The Real Race

The day after I asked Julie and Sue about running a full marathon, Stephen and another friend, Jim, told me they had signed up for the Columbus full. Several other friends had also signed up for the October race. "You'll have company on Saturdays," Stephen said, referring to the long runs that would take much of the day.

I looked at the schedule. The weekday runs were only a mile longer than those at the end of the half schedule. Maybe, I thought. Maybe.

On that eleven-mile run, Julie said she schedules an hour and a half massage after her long runs. Despite having gone through four massage therapists, I scheduled massages the day after each Saturday run and daydreamed about running longer.

Pain and mental agony marred my next run with Morgan. We missed a turn, my ankle ached, and I'd overdressed. Afterward, my ankle swelled for the first time in many months. Depression surfaced—not the stay-in-bed-all-day kind, but a general heaviness in my limbs and mind. Thoughts of the full had excited me, and I felt let-down. Some people can handle roller coasters. My emotions require a tight rein. I told myself the marathon would be there when I was ready. I wrote in my log, "I'm crazy to think about a full. I can't take the pain." I wasn't sure I could even run the upcoming half.

Like a yo-yo, an up followed the down. During a few pain-free runs, the faces of everyone training for the full arose in my mind. Could I turn myself into a morning person and finish each run before it became too hot? Should I give up social media? Should I take up weight training and swimming? Should I cut my carbs? Thoughts flared like trick birthday candles. As soon as I snuffed out one, another flared.

After our last long run before the Cap City Half, our pace group went to breakfast. Over eggs and coffee, we planned our carb-loading and expo visit. Inevitably, talk turned to the October full. Race-week taper tension, blended with images of the 26.2 sticker, made it difficult to talk myself down. The upcoming half looked like a stepping stone.

***

At the Cap City Expo and on my way to the race, I remembered the previous year when I'd "only" done the quarter. This year I was doing the "whole" half—the "real" race.

On race morning, Jeff, the Tall Guy, yelled "Have a great race!" into the boom box. We put our bags in the truck, walked to the corrals, and visited the porta potties. I excused my way through the packed corral from the east side of Marconi to the west side, trying to find Ed. Five minutes before the start, he appeared. He'd been taking photos. I squeezed out to greet him, but when I returned, my pace group had left. I frantically searched the crowd, but the mass of people pushed me toward the start line. I waved to Ed and began to run.

For a few strides, I listened to my metronome to get my cadence. As usual, I'd started out faster than I'd intended, but it felt comfortable, so I continued at that pace. Between miles one and two, I caught up with friends. At the water stop, I pulled ahead. Bands played. Fans cheered. And I felt no pain.

Olentangy River Road stretched on and on, but I looked forward to seeing Ed at Olentangy and Lane. I passed beneath the Woody Hayes Drive overpass early, so I called Ed to let him know I was ahead of schedule. He was at Schottenstein Arena, getting petitions signed. He had tickets to see POTUS and FLOTUS. When I approached, he stood in front of the arena, waving his clipboard. I blew kisses and turned away, conflicted about not waiting to hug and kiss him.

At mile five, Jeff bicycled past, traveling the course to support MIT. He noticed my scowl and said, "Take it easy. It's still a long way." He didn't know I was only blue about not stopping for Ed. Otherwise, I felt strong. Seeing Jeff lifted my spirits. I wasn't alone.

As I continued down Lane, I hadn't completely shaken my sadness at not getting to kiss Ed. Then I saw Andy and the Front Runner running store crew cheering. His high-five helped too. Another boost came near Lane and High, when I recognized Matthew, a friend, playing trombone in a band. His eyes grew wide, and he cheered when he saw me. He didn't know I ran.

The spectator-lined, two-and-a-half-mile stretch of High Street on campus wore on me. But seeing the same raggedy guy who'd been at the previous half on his bike with a boom box blaring the theme from *Chariots of Fire* gave me a lift.

In the Short North, I clapped for the person riding a bicycle in a purple velvet dress. Cars waiting to turn had lined up in the left lane. A guy had his arm out his window, so I high-fived him. In a chain reaction, people rolled down their windows and I high-fived them all.

Ahead of pace, I thought about a PR (personal record). But when we turned onto Long, the wind whipped my face. Folks complained about the humidity, but I didn't notice it. On Washington, headed toward the freeway, I recognized the swinging ponytail of my friend Heather, the "real runner" Morgan and I had raced with nearly a year ago. She was now pregnant and walking. She welcomed a hug.

I ran ahead to catch a pace group friend and we crossed the freeway into German Village. The brick streets in Schiller Park hurt my feet, but soon we caught another friend. It was turning into a party.

At our pre-race dinner, Sue had suggested I speed up at mile nine, but I'd forgotten. On High Street, at mile twelve, I told my friend I was picking it up. She sped up too. My left Achilles objected. I began heel-striking to protect it. When I saw the finish, I yelled, "Let's go!" I relaxed my whole body and sprinted. MIT folks, including Sarah, the marathoner who had impressed me with her blue full medal, yelled, "Go, Nita!" I smiled for the photographers.

Kelley, now very pregnant, had volunteered. She gave me my medal. I hugged and thanked her, remembering our first half marathon together.

My ankles stung and my knee ached, so I went to the medical tent for ice. Dr. Bright, the race medical director, said my ChiRunning stride probably wasn't natural yet and tweaked my Achilles. Kelley found me wrapped in ice. We walked to her car, and she drove me back to the hotel. I laughed at how people kept appearing. I'd never been alone.

I'd beaten my personal record by sixteen minutes. My ankle swelled, my knee hurt, my quads burned, and it was absolutely worth it.

***

For three days after the race, my ankle remained swollen and my Achilles sore. My spirits sank. I iced, took ibuprofen, gently stretched, slept, and cried, convinced I'd permanently injured myself.

After four days, the swelling went down and the pain subsided, so I tried a two-mile run with the dog. In the race photos, I was either heel-striking or it looked like I was walking. Now, I slowed and leaned from my center of gravity. I kept my shoulders back and my legs under me. I had no idea what correct form was supposed to feel like, but I had no pain during the run and celebrated not being permanently damaged.

Meanwhile, my friends continued signing up for the 2012 Columbus full marathon. I imagined saying, "I'm training for a full," going for long runs in the heat of summer surrounded by friends and putting the coveted 26.2 sticker on my car.

Julie and Sue had finished their races and intended to sign up for Columbus, five months away. Our previous coaches were taking time off, so Julie became a coach. Jennifer, another friend who also intended to run the full, stepped up to be the other. While I still worried that my wonky ankle or my cycling moods might keep me from achieving my goal, knowing I could run with them tipped the scale.

Ed and I agreed on a plan: I'd sign up, set an intention, and train. Then I'd see what happened.

In my office, with Morgan snoring on the floor beside me, I had trouble steadying the mouse enough to click "register" on the

Columbus Marathon website. When the confirmation email popped into my inbox, I squealed and Morgan barked. That made it official.

CHAPTER 21

A Real Runner

"I'm training for a FULL marathon!" I giddily chanted to myself as I drove to the first MIT session of the new season. Our pace group conversed in early-morning grunts and shrugs until Jeff, the Tall Guy, motioned for us to start. It was only May and barely seven in the morning, but sweat dampened my armpits before we hit the trailhead. Giddiness gave way to letdown. This was not momentous. It was just another run.

A few folks with hangovers complained. Thank goodness I hadn't had a hangover in more than two decades. Then I thought, "Maybe ordinary is perfect." Each week of longer miles would bring new challenges, but mostly, it was a normal Saturday on the Olentangy Trail. Anti-climactic was good! My smile lasted for the rest of the run.

The schedule said six miles, but the veteran full marathoner coaches decided to only run four with the halfs. I told Coach Julie I would run two more with the vicious carnivore at home. She scolded me, worried I would overtrain and injure myself. At home, I settled for one more. I slowly circled Ed and the dog to the end of the street. Then the dog and I slow-jogged the rest of the mile.

***

The first "marathon" was run in 490 BC by the soldier Pheidippides, who ran approximately twenty-five miles from Marathon, Greece, to Athens to announce the defeat of the Persians. After making his proclamation, he collapsed and died.

The marathon distance remained twenty-five miles until 1908 when, at the request of the British Queen Alexandra, the course was extended. She wanted the race to start on the lawn of Windsor Castle, so the royal youngsters could watch from the nursery, and to finish at the royal box in Olympic Stadium. That made the race twenty-six miles and 385 yards. The marathon distance has been 26.2 miles ever since.

I hoped the marathon wouldn't kill me.

***

Two days after that first full marathon training run, the dog and I did five miles. I ran fast on my somewhat still swollen ankle, trying to hit the ground midfoot. I thought I might finally be getting it.

A mile from home, daydreaming about the marathon, I tripped. As I fell, I thought, "I'll catch myself."

WHAM! I landed on right hand, right elbow, and left knee before my chest slammed into the concrete, reverberating with sharp pain. I skidded off the sidewalk onto a neighbor's lawn and lay there, trying to catch my breath. My first thought was that I'd had a heart attack and passed out. Then I remembered the sensation of flying. A tiny lip between sidewalk slabs had caught my shoe.

I noticed a pair of tennis shoes and rolled over. A tall young man with grass stains on the knees of his jeans stared down. "Ma'am?" Someone yelled, "Should I call 911?" The young man helped me sit up.

Then I remembered Morgan, who was sniffing the grass near the street. The man grabbed his leash and two other men, also in grass-stained clothes, came over. These handsome, sweaty young men called me "Ma'am" as if I were their grandmother. Embarrassed, I chided myself for running on the sidewalk when other runners had warned against it. But I also thought, "I took a tumble and lived. I'm really a runner." Then I remembered to stop my Garmin.

The owner of the house, a man in his seventies, approached. Two of the men scattered back across the yard, but the first stayed, still holding Morgan's leash. The owner asked, "Do you need a ride home?" I shook my head. "Just help me to my feet." They took my arms and I stood, painfully.

But I was shaking, hard. They didn't let go. A few tentative deep breaths confirmed that my lungs still worked. Morgan panted nervously. I centered myself, noticing the power in my belly and my feet solid beneath me. "I'll be okay. They're just scrapes," I said. They each loosened their grip and I wobbled, then straightened. The owner told me his name, which I promptly forgot. I told him mine and thanked them.

As I walked toward home, I told myself that I was okay. Ed would kiss my boo-boos and put on Band-Aids. At the end of the block, I began a slow jog. That went well, so I continued. Soon Morgan and I were running again. "I'll be sore tomorrow, but I'll be fine," I told the dog.

At home, I washed the patch of skin on my left thigh that looked as if I'd slid into home plate, applied antibiotic ointment, and covered it. Ed hugged and kissed me. That night at our recovery group, friends examined my bandages, hugged me, and murmured encouraging words. I said it was no big deal but felt like a badass. At home, I took ibuprofen and went to bed.

The next morning, when I rolled over, knife-like pain stabbed my ribcage. I researched "broken ribs." Treatment comprised ibuprofen or stronger pain pills I won't take due to my tendency toward addiction. A medical website recommended deep breaths, making yourself cough every hour, and stretching gently throughout the day. Running that weekend hurt a little, but not terribly. What hurt was lying down, bending over, and getting up in the morning. Breathing sometimes hurt, too.

I had hoped to start weight training, but that had to wait, since I could barely lift my book bag. My right hand, the one I mouse with, was tender too. The road rash healed nicely, but my ribs remained achy. An x-ray showing nothing and a doctor okaying me to run would reassure me, but if a doctor told me not to run, I'd have to say, "Too late." I continued to heal by not lifting anything and not falling again. That was actual advice on the internet: "Under no circumstances should you fall again if you have broken ribs." Um, well. I hadn't intended to fall in the first place!

When I still hurt two weeks later, I went to urgent care. The x-ray was negative. He said broken ribs rarely show on x-rays right away, so it was good I had waited.

My runs following the fall were a forced exercise in mindfulness. I didn't take ibuprofen before a run because I feared the drug might mask another injury. Getting the x-ray allowed me to stop worrying about punctured lungs, but the mild pain still caused brain chatter. When I found my rhythm and tilted my pelvis to allow my rib cage to expand, it no longer hurt to breathe. But the occasional jarring step sent a jolt of pain through my chest, causing me to think I was having a heart attack. When I remembered I'd recently fallen, I'd chant "It's just your ribs" until I calmed down.

***

In the days following the half and before I'd fallen, my ankle had swelled again. Sprinting to the finish hadn't been worth the seconds it saved. Nothing hurt while I ran, but after, if I sat for very long, the blood pooled and my ankle grew tender.

I continued icing and wore compression hose in the evening. I sometimes wore them to bed, but it was summer, and I am a middle-aged woman with hot flashes. I put my feet up often and, at the computer, swung my leg over an open file-cabinet drawer.

My previous experience with the ankle told me the swelling and pain would pass. My ankle had swollen when I first started running but grew accustomed to the movement and the swelling stopped. Now it needed to become familiar with additional miles and faster, short runs. Plus, the summer heat caused everything to swell.

Instead of going to a doctor for the dreaded MRI, anti-anxiety medication, nightmares before and after, and the possibility of being told not to run, I continued to see my chiropractor, wrapped my ankle in an ace bandage, did toe-points and ankle circles, took arnica pills, and applied arnica cream. These wouldn't cure it, but kept it loose and reduced the swelling.

I also shortened my weekday runs.

I had my first period in about four months and wondered if hormones impacted my ankle. I so wished there were a running doctor who prescribed herbs, massage, and gentle movement the way my chiropractor did.

I wanted to tell the overweight ankle surgeon who said running was bad for you to shove it. Deep inside, however, I was still afraid he was right. I wanted to believe the body could heal itself. The only way to find out was to continue to run.

***

Ten days after I fell, Mr. Dawg and I ran our second Pet Promise Rescue Run. The two-lap course was again punctuated by water dishes, baby pools, and dog poop containers. The race didn't start until ten thirty in the morning and attendance was down, possibly due to the high temperatures. Mr. Dawg and I started too fast and my ribs still hurt. I was grateful he stopped to drink at each bucket. He peed in one bucket, so I kicked it over.

Many folks walked due to the heat. Between the second and third mile, Mr. Dawg, panting hard, stepped into a baby pool and lay down. I scooped handfuls of water onto his head and neck, prepared to stay there as long as he needed.

As I contemplated my first DNF ("did not finish" or "did nothing fatal"), his breathing returned to normal. A woman with a greyhound trotted past and Morgan leapt to his feet. He gave me a disgusted eyeroll when I pulled him back and held firm. I did not want him to overheat again. Near the finish, I let him trot. Then I guided him into one of the waiting baby pools to cool down. When he stopped panting, I let him drink. Then we headed to the air-conditioned car.

***

The following Monday, Memorial Day, marked my second running of the five-miler through our neighborhood. Despite my still-aching ribs and the heat, I was excited to meet, in person, some runners from the online group, the "Dead Runners Society" (DRS).

The DRS listserv took its name from the 1989 movie, *Dead Poets Society*. The group motto, "Carpe Viam," loosely translated, means "Seize the Road!" People from around the globe have attended their "World Conference." Our small Memorial Day gathering was what the group calls a "Dead Encounter." As my experience with running grew, I'd moved from the "Penguins" beginner forum to sharing "Obligatory Run Note" entries with the Deads via email. I'd only recently learned that a "Dead" couple lived just one block away.

That morning, I met the couple and another Columbus Dead by the flagpole near the fire station where the race began. The couple looked like the marathoners they are—trim and muscular. They travel the country to run different races throughout the year. In 2011, they ran fourteen marathons. The other woman was also trim and fit. She was recovering from an injury and would run/walk, the method championed by Olympian Jeff Galloway. I'd worried these DRS "real runners" might judge me, but they were friendly and warm.

At the gun, the couple took off. I stayed with the solo woman. When it was time for her to walk, understanding the runner's code to each run your own race, she motioned for me to go ahead. I want to be loyal and enjoyed her company, but also wanted to PR. My mind went back and forth. I sped ahead, looked back, and she waved. Eventually, I stopped looking back.

In the second mile, a deer bolted across the road, waving his white tail high. On an out-and-back part of the course, the woman of the Dead couple waved. She had a good ten-minute lead on me, and her husband was ahead of her.

At the block near our house, Ed, Morgan and our neighbors were waiting. The two red-headed girls who lived on the corner, whose father, Luke, was also running, cheered as I climbed the hill. I picked up my pace and Ed snapped a flattering picture while Morgan barked and bounced, indignant at being left behind.

At the next water stop, I drank one cup and poured a second over my head. Neighbors on ladders held spray hoses to refresh us as we ran beneath them. My ribs hurt, but I reminded myself I'd paid perfectly

good money to run through the neighborhood I can run any day
for free.

It was ninety degrees when the Dead couple and Ed greeted me at
the finish. I had PR'd by six seconds. I slugged down two bottles of
water and searched for shade.

We cheered as the run/walker Dead approached the finish. But her
shoe caught the finish-line timing mat, and she fell hard on her wrist.
Emergency personnel approached, then swept her into the building.
Her wrist was sprained, not broken, but I knew how sore she'd be in
the coming weeks.

The women in my age group beat me by many minutes. Ed and
I clapped for every winner, especially a woman in her seventies
who won her age group. I told Ed, "That's who I want to be when I
grow up."

After the race, I took a three-hour nap. That night I went to bed early
and slept until noon. The physical exertion and social interaction of
two races so close together sapped my energy for much of that week. I
worried that I lacked the stamina for a marathon.

***

The first Saturday of June, our MIT pace group included twenty half
marathoners and six training for the full. Trail banter distracted me
from my still-sore ribs. The half marathoners were running three.
We "fulls" "only" had six miles and were bubbly. We ran with the
halfs for one and a half miles, until they stopped to turn around. I
shuddered with anxiety and joy when the six of us continued without
them. I'd felt a similar rush when I'd run with the fulls last season,
but now, instead of just running a mile with them, then running back
alone, I was going all the way.

On our way back, a man yelled "bike back" to let us know a bike was
about to pass. We tucked in to run single file. Then he yelled, "Punch
it!" I hugged the edge of the trail expecting a group to fly by. Instead,
a little boy, maybe four or five, burst past on a bike with training
wheels, head down, pedaling for all he was worth. I laughed so hard I
nearly fell again. Our group claimed "Punch it!" as our motto.

***

A few days later, I attended a New Balance "Good Form Running Clinic." My face flushed with pride as I introduced myself and said I was training for the Columbus full. I was easily the oldest, heaviest person there.

I was well-versed in running technique lingo, having implemented ChiRunning form focuses for more than a year. I'd read *Pose Running,* attended several Natural Running clinics by Newton Shoes, read *Born to Run,* and tried to practice the techniques prescribed by Caballo Blanco as summarized by Chris McDougall.

I knew most of the answers to the instructor's questions, chimed in about my portable metronome, and cheerfully showed how I'd learned to reset my posture on the run. My enthusiasm may have annoyed the other participants, but as a true believer, I didn't care. When I focused on form, my body hurt less.

The instructor gave us drills to help us experience each of the four aspects of form. For posture, align the feet, keep knees loose, do the yoga Mountain Pose to tilt the pelvis and loosen the shoulders. For midfoot strike, march in place on the midfoot. For cadence, the goal is rapid foot turnover, ideally at least 180 beats per minute. With my metronome, I'd progressed from 150 to 170. And, finally, for lean, get the right posture, lean forward from your ankles until your toes curl, then pick up one foot and go.

I found the marching in place (to feel the midfoot strike) and the Mountain Pose "posture reset" (to feel the posture) especially helpful. This was the first time I'd sensed these in my body, as opposed to just having the idea in my head.

Before class, they videotaped us. The instructor complimented me on how my head stayed on a level plane as I ran. I didn't bounce. My arms swung well, but my hand crossed in front of my body and my upper body twisted. My cadence was the best in the class, and I had a decent lean. Sadly, I was landing on my heels. My form had improved, but the heel-striking and over-striding discouraged me. I wanted that midfoot strike.

The workshop reminded me to use form as my object of meditation during each run. When Mr. Dawg stopped, which was often, I did the drills to remind my body how proper form feels. I used my metronome and looked at the Good Form Running Clinic cheat sheet, determined to improve.

***

Then Sara, our former pace coach, the same coach whose mother had died of a heart attack, developed deep vein thrombosis and a pulmonary embolism. Deep vein thrombosis (DVT) commonly afflicts people who travel by plane or who sit for long periods. The blood pools and coagulates.

Long-distance runners are also prone to the condition. Running causes the resting heart rate to drop, which slows blood circulation and promotes coagulation. I was a long-distance runner who sat a lot, as well as a hypochondriac. After her incident, I compulsively checked my legs. My calf hurt. It looked red, but that might have been sunburn. I took a baby aspirin which, as far as I know does nothing for DVT, and hoped for the best.

I sent Sara baby animal photos, jokes and motivational sayings to cheer her. Mostly, I sent them to distract myself. I begged the Universe to let her recover. She would, but it would be slow and painful. She blogged about her experience as she recuperated. When I read these posts, I scanned my legs for symptoms, found them, took another baby aspirin, and talked myself out of going to the ER. Later I learned that the symptoms of DVT are like those of varicose veins, except that DVT pain is more severe. Since I have varicose veins, I told myself they caused the pain and continued running. I had a marathon to train for.

***

A few days after our full marathon group encountered the boy on the training-wheel bicycle, we tried to recreate the scene. We remembered, "Punch it!" but not the boy's name, which the father had also yelled.

"Punch it, John?" No. "Punch it, Roger?"

The following week, we did seven miles. Stephen and I paired off to talk about dogs, politics, and weather. I told him about the cute little boy.

Cyclists and runners filled the trail. When Stephen and I were deep in conversation, I saw the same little boy, followed by a man I guessed to be his father, approaching. I got so excited, I nearly fell down the embankment into the river. I righted myself, pointed to the boy and called out, "Did you tell him to 'Punch it!' last Saturday on the trail?" The man laughed and nodded. We stood in the trail while I told him our running group adopted that as our motto.

"What's his name?"

"Jake," the father said proudly. I thanked him for solving our mystery.

Later that day I messaged the others. "Punch it, Jake!" was our marathon slogan.

CHAPTER 22

Roller Coaster

After our pace coach had the pulmonary embolism, calf pain became my constant companion. Instead of getting it checked, I obsessed. During runs, when I focused on form, my calves didn't hurt, but afterward, they were painful. I looked over the pace coach's symptoms. Was it a sharp pain? A cramp? Was my leg swollen or were my muscles growing from intense workouts? Should I go to the urgent care? Not today. Maybe tomorrow.

***

Typical of central Ohio, the middle of June through the middle of August was stifling. I took water for the dog, but sometimes we wound up stopping to rest in the shade. I'm not a morning person, so often started late. On the hottest days, I left the pouting dog behind, making for a lonely, but quicker, run since I didn't have to stop for him to pee.

When MIT cancelled our Saturday run due to lightning, Julie, Sue, and I ran on Sunday. It was still humid from the storm and trees were down. Bunnies hopping along the trail and a raccoon in an overturned trash can at Antrim startled us. We declared it "Nature Day."

Later that month, MIT cancelled the Saturday run again due to predicted heat. I needed to clear my head, so I planned to at least run four miles. I rose before dawn and read Dead Runner's Society emails while the sun came up. It was already seventy-five degrees with ninety percent humidity. Our slow run through what felt like warm fog took an extra half-hour because Morgan and I stopped frequently to drink and cool down. I drank two eight-ounce bottles of homemade Gatorade and Morgan emptied a twenty-ounce pink handheld of water. That day's high of ninety-nine degrees made it the hottest July day that year.

I missed our MIT ten-miler, so ran that without Mr. Dawg, since it was again too hot for him. The image of him staring longingly through the kitchen window tortured me. Each bit of trash on the street infuriated me. I was actually just pissed because it was so hot. Eventually I distracted myself by focusing on form. Afterward, I took Morgan for a single mile in the shade as penance.

If thunderstorms threatened, the dog and I did one-mile laps through the ravine. I left my bottle and Morgan's dish by the street so we could stop and sip as we passed the house. We improvised to make it through.

Early in the summer, I searched for shoes less cushioned than the Newtons but softer than the Merrell Pace Gloves. Merrell Bare Access Arcs were comfortable, but the heel showed wear after only a few runs and the bottoms of my feet hurt. I tried wearing cushioned socks, but my Newtons were more comfortable. I wasn't ready to graduate to the Bare Access Arcs. I bought the newest model of Newtons in a perky teal.

***

I'd grown bored with my metronome. Listening to *Three Non Joggers* helped distract me from my negative mental chatter, but also distracted me from form and cadence. I unconsciously matched my foot turnover to the show's music, which was rarely near 180 beats per minute.

Googling "music with 180 b.p.m. (beats per minute)" revealed several prepared playlists. Most had lyrics, which I find stressful. My mind latches onto the words and won't let go. I prefer classical, smooth jazz, or even elevator renditions of popular songs. I downloaded two Acoustic Alchemy songs with close to 180 b.p.m. On my next run, I used those to get my rhythm, listening with just one earbud. With only two songs, I grew bored, but whenever I sensed my foot turnover slowing, I turned them on, and my cadence rose to tempo.

***

Despite the overall benefits of running, my emotions continued to cycle. Some mornings I woke frightened by voices outside the bedroom window when no one was there. Whenever I saw a stranger sitting in a car on our street, I assumed the person was casing our house to break in after we left. Other days I shopped uncontrollably for running clothes, then grimaced at the stack of price tags accumulating on the dresser.

During one run in a torrential downpour, the dog and I startled a mother raccoon and two babies hiding in the storm sewer. Another day I wondered as I wore my water belt if passersby thought, "Look at her! She's running so far she has to carry water." More points toward my badass merit badge. The dog shook his head. He thought they were thinking we were silly to run far enough to need water.

When the dog and I happened upon my cousin Mark, whose company was painting a house in my neighborhood, he exclaimed "Look at you!" as I trotted over for a hug. Morgan napped in the shade while Mark and I talked. The impressed look on his face made me feel like a real runner.

By this time, I had amassed a small collection of race medals. Ed mounted a display rack on the wall in the bedroom I use for an office. When I felt down, I looked at the shiny medals.

Running helped my emotional stability, but I continued to struggle with decisions. I had a schedule, but choosing what time of day or day of the week to run, which route to take, or what clothes to wear tormented me. Some days, unable to decide, I sat in the house, playing computer solitaire. I put off running until the heat of the day, then was miserable as the dog and I sweated it out. Other days I postponed to the next day, only to sit again for hours, plagued by anxiety. It took tremendous effort to get going, but on the streets I felt better.

In the middle of July, I ran ten miles alone in brutal heat. There had been three landscape companies on our street, and since I couldn't force myself to leave the house until they were gone, it was too warm to take Morgan. I stopped to stretch and sat on a wall near the park to drink water and rest. Each time I began to run, the scene of me skidding across the sidewalk after I fell looped in my mind. I sang the "Happy Little Cell" song to block the image. But my legs grew heavy. Ten miles wasn't even close to a marathon. I couldn't possibly run two and a half times that. I reminded myself, "You don't have to do it today." Back home, I showered, wrapped my swollen ankle in a compression bandage, and curled up with Morgan for a nap. I woke calmer, my body filled with the warm, post-run glow.

In the heat of July, a few of us from MIT ran the Color Run. The point is to get covered with colored cornstarch and look like a rainbow. I bought a white running skirt, but when I tested it beforehand, it chafed. When I showered, raw skin met water in a vicious sting. I tossed the skirt in the donation box.

The race wasn't timed, so my friends and I rolled on the ground to get more color on our clothes. Ed waved from the porch of the Victorian mansion that housed his office as we ran by. Some people like obstacle races where you crawl through mud or under barbed wire and jump over fire. Not me. Give me unicorns and rainbows. My inner three-year-old danced. By the end, I was covered in color, but I'd worn a tech shirt instead of the recommended cotton, so the color washed out.

***

I was jealous when people who'd started with our pace group moved to faster groups. I could work on speed or distance, not both. And I had things backward. I should have been running the Saturday long runs more slowly than the weekly ones. But even though we full marathoners were slower than the halfs, the Saturday runs were faster.

As the length of the runs extended, my pace slowed by over a minute per mile. Julie and Sue experienced the same thing. They'd each run a full marathon the spring before and wanted to PR. I simply wanted to finish, but feared getting swept. We wouldn't win the race, but I wanted that 26.2 sticker. I also hoped to stay with them so I wouldn't have to run alone.

The beginner marathon schedule didn't include speed work, so I made up my own. Some days, during shorter runs, I ran fast and hard. I liked PR'ing a route in the neighborhood. But Morgan lagged on these speedy runs. Since I preferred running with the dog and the dog wouldn't be able to run forever, I usually skipped the speed work.

One day, when Morgan and I were running up a hill near our house, a pit bull boxer mix dashed into the street after Morgan. I yelled, dragged Morgan away, and sped off. The dog didn't follow. A block away, with my heart still pounding, I told Morgan, "That's not the kind of speed work I meant!"

When I caught myself referring to seven miles as "short," I laughed at how my perspective had changed. Ten miles gave way to twelve. By mid-summer, we were running a half marathon every weekend.

***

One July day, Mr. Dawg and I ran through our neighborhood in tense air the consistency of warm soup. The sky clouded, threatening rain. The heat seemed to bring out the dogs. A chocolate Lab stuck half its body out the back window of a passing SUV, barking and biting the air. Minutes later, two other Labs on leashes, one yellow and one black, grumbled at us, their owner seemingly oblivious.

A few blocks from there, a loose German Shepherd mix in a black harness crept toward us with no owner in sight. He eyed us warily, fluffed his fur and circled. I slowed. "Good dog. Good dog," I said as he approached with his ears back and head down. I intended to squirt water in his eyes if he attacked, but I was shaking so hard I almost dropped the bottle.

When the dog closed in and tried to sniff Morgan's behind, Morgan growled, then let out a guttural woof so deep and loud that the loose dog and I both jumped. The other dog leaned away. I slowly backed up and only turned around once the dog was out of sight. We sprinted up a steep hill on pure adrenaline, then I collapsed in the street at the top and wrapped my arms around Morgan's smooth neck. I cried until I calmed down.

I wished all the dogs we encountered were like the Chihuahuas and the beagles. Some days the Chihuahuas ran loose in the yard of their corner lot while their lady sat in her lawn chair smoking cigarettes. She often complimented me on my bright shoes. The white and black Chihuahua would race to the edge of the street and bark while running along the curb into the neighbor's yard. I'm wary of the Chihuahuas since I've known several who bite, but this dog never ventured into the street. The black one also barked but didn't run. If they were indoors, they yapped and bounced harmlessly against their bay window. Further down the street, the friendly beagles often bayed at us from behind the safety of their chain-link fence.

Having recovered from our encounter with the grumpy dog, Morgan and I jogged home. In the house, I lay on the floor with him. I scratched his back and thanked him for protecting us. We were both discovering our hidden strengths.

Shortly after the Good Form Running Clinic, I'd begun doing posture resets, where you raise your arms over your head, then put your hands together in Mountain Pose. Some days the posture resets were too awkward and embarrassing to do while carrying the dog leash. I ran during the cooler mornings and evenings when others also ran, so I didn't have the streets to myself. People were in their houses potentially (but probably not) watching, and runners, bicyclists, and walkers of all ages were out. I imagined the teens laughing at me even without my doing posture resets, so I abandoned them except when alone. Other days, depending on the level of my mental health and self-conscious self-centeredness, I did posture resets anyway.

***

Stephen and I both missed the first fourteen-mile group run. At six thirty on a Monday morning I paced the high school parking lot, waiting for him to arrive so we could make up the miles together. I was certain fourteen miles would either kill me from boredom or flare my wonky ankle and force my training to a stop.

Across the parking lot, a middle-aged man with a gray beard pulled up in a rusty Chevy sedan. Not Stephen. The stranger stared from behind his wheel. I climbed back in my station wagon and turned on classical radio trying not to stare back. Eventually Stephen arrived, but I was convinced the man would follow us.

Stephen and I ran the wooded trail to the north, over the bridge and into the meadow along the Olentangy River. Dew rose off the ground, and the previous day's rain greened the trees and grass. Gratitude for the scenery flooding my senses, and for Stephen telling story after story to pass the time, filled my heart. I only looked over my shoulder a few times to check for the man in the car.

We took our first bathroom break near the gazebo at Worthington Hills. We're both over fifty, so neither objected when the other wanted to use the facilities. At Antrim, we stopped for another potty break. The sun sat low and mist rose from the lake. South of Antrim, between the river and Route 315, the traffic was so loud Stephen had to shout, but he didn't stop talking. In half a mile, the trail turned toward the river. Trees muted the noise.

I love and hate the shady trail between Antrim Lake and Henderson Road. It has few landmarks, so it seems endless. But it's also tree-lined and lush. Today, with Stephen talking, it passed quickly. At a little bench, I thought, "I'd like to lie down," then remembered the man in the parking lot. There was no sign of him.

We headed back toward the school, and Stephen retrieved water bottles he had stashed under a tree. My hands were so weak I had trouble opening mine. Stephen doesn't like to stop for long. I dawdle, so this was good practice.

Over the Henderson bridge, back down the hill, back under the bridge, and into the woods we ran. The trail looks different coming from the opposite direction. I appreciated the change.

The sun now sparkled on Antrim Lake. As I remarked how beautiful it was, someone on a bike blew past, nearly knocking me down. The next small hill left both of us breathing hard. We had picked up the pace as we closed in on the finish. Stephen had stopped talking.

At the top, Stephen gasped, "I'm trying to get some semblance of form back."

"I lost mine six miles ago," I panted. I checked my cadence with my metronome. It was slow, so I picked it up. My knee hurt, so I tilted my pelvis, lifted my feet, and kept my knees bent while trying to relax. Soon the pain went away.

At thirteen miles, Stephen said, "Congrats on a half marathon!" At 13.2, the longest distance I'd ever run, he congratulated me again.

My head swam and my legs dragged as we plodded wordlessly up the long hill toward the school. At the speed bumps, I ran toward the space in the middle so I wouldn't have to lift my feet. I kept telling myself, "We're almost there." At the stop sign, my watch read 13.7 and Stephen's 13.9. "Need to go flat?" he asked, already knowing the answer. We continued until my watch read fourteen. Then we walked around the mostly-empty parking lot to cool down. My whole body ached. The stranger I'd worried about earlier was gone.

At home, I rolled "The Stick," a long pole with flat white beads, over my legs to smooth out the knots. I didn't take an ice bath. I'd read an article questioning their efficacy. Besides, they're so unpleasant. I don't have a foam roller. The stick hurt enough. The next day, my ankle was swollen. I wrapped and elevated it. Still, fourteen miles amazed me. Two years before, I couldn't even run around the block.

***

The Saturday long runs in the full marathon training schedule had begun at four miles. Each week for three weeks, the schedule added one mile to the run. The fourth week, we "fell back" to lower mileage for one Saturday to allow our bodies to recover. The week after Stephen and I ran fourteen, Julie and I missed the group ten-mile "fallback" run. On Sunday, we made up the miles easily on a trail busy with folks enjoying sunny but cool weather. We planned our marathon-day strategy of positioning friends to cheer us along the final miles of the race.

The following Saturday, our group ran the second fourteen-miler in Westerville, through the neighborhood and onto the Genoa Trail. The sun sparkled through the trees onto the trail and pond. A little bridge on Hoover Preserve Trail didn't scare me at all, and a good-sized hill challenged us. We shared funny stories. Jennifer said, "An acorn fell out of my panties this morning!" Her son had collected a pine cone and an acorn on a hike, and they wound up in their laundry. She'd found the pine cone, but not the acorn, until this morning when it flew out of her underpants as she put them on. We found it extra funny because Jennifer was our fashion plate, always dressed in stylish workout gear. Plus, she worked in the underwear industry and could identify the brand and style of any bra made.

On the way out, Stephen and I lagged together. When we turned around, I stayed with the group. Stephen was doing "time on his feet" instead of distance. When he hit four hours, he started to walk. We finished without him and hung around the Ohio Health building to talk. Ten minutes passed, and still no Stephen. I went back out to find him. He'd become dizzy and sat down on the sidewalk. He told us not to worry, that he would be fine after food and a nap. Later he texted to say he had called his doctor.

Stephen's health concerned me, but I was amazed at how much less fatigue I felt than after our first fourteen-mile run. This time I'd focused on form, used the metronome, and done several posture resets. The Newtons also helped. Still, I couldn't imagine twelve additional miles. When I told Julie this, she asked, "But could you do two more?" I said "Yes," and Julie said, "That's all you have to do next week."

CHAPTER 23

Sore Feet

As the searing summer days wore on, even the "short" midweek "easy" runs, now six miles, challenged me. My left knee continued to ache and my left hip started to hurt. I hadn't magically become a morning person, so it was often too hot to take Mr. Dawg. Even if I took him, I grew bored. His conversational skills had not improved over our years of running together.

It was also dry. The cracked ground reminded me of suicidal days I'd spent in the New Mexico desert, years before. But I did what I'd learned in meditation and writing. Keep showing up. I always felt better after.

***

For the following week's eighteen-miler, Jennifer, Julie, and I started in the dark at five thirty in the morning to get a few miles in before the group. As coaches, they had to run with the halfs, then go back out to finish the full marathon mileage. We ran through a Worthington neighborhood. Even with street lights illuminating the sidewalk, when a dog barked, I jumped so hard I nearly knocked Julie down. It took a minute before we all realized the dog was in a house, not chasing us.

Then it rained. Not hard, but enough to soak my shoes and socks by mile four. Some of the halfs complained and I was not in the mood to listen. The heavier my mind, the heavier my legs. Plus, eighteen is just difficult. Around four miles, I decided I wouldn't make it. I couldn't settle into my stride.

Julie suggested a running mantra. At meditation retreats, I'd learned about the benefits of these repeated phrases. I whispered, "Run strong, run free." My legs still ached, but my attitude sucked less.

Julie reminded me that running is ninety percent mental. Later she added, "And the rest is mental!"

When we dropped off the half marathoners, we fulls had twelve and a half more to run. I'm not sure who suggested that running seven miles south, then back, would achieve this, but none of us were alert enough to catch it until someone's watch hit eighteen and we were still three-quarters of a mile from our cars. This was not the first time (nor would it be the last) that we failed at "math while running."

At home, I looked at the bottoms of my Newtons. The edge was worn off where I'd been heel-striking. I checked my running logs. No wonder I hurt! The Newtons had logged nearly five hundred miles.

***

On Labor Day, I took Morgan for a muggy three-mile run before Ed and I drove to Ann Arbor, home of the University of *ichigan, the arch-rivals of Ohio State University. (Buckeyes don't use the "M" word). My legs were still tired from the eighteen-miler, but I didn't want to leave the dog without a run.

While Ed attended a conference on guardianship, his latest volunteer adventure, I ran. I wasn't brave enough to wear Ohio State gear around the *ichigan campus, so I wore unmarked clothes. On the route, I darted under a bridge that was under construction, heart racing.

Afterward, I noticed a new pain in my left foot. Ed said it looked like a pinprick. I worried it was a stress fracture, but it felt more like a sting. Perhaps it was the deadly brown recluse spider. I iced my foot and the pain subsided. I took my shoe off several times to examine it and took a lot of ibuprofen. I imagined pain on the next day's miles as I sat in the hot tub. I couldn't run a marathon with a swollen foot.

In the morning, I found the Ann Arbor Arboretum, despite fearing I wouldn't, and ran five slow, hilly miles. On this, my first trail run, I saw three types of squirrels: gray, red, and coal black, plus a hawk. But with two bathroom breaks and the slow pace, I returned almost forty-five minutes after I'd planned. When I walked through the hotel door, the strain on Ed's face reminded me I should have called. It was the same look he'd had years before when, the day after I'd been released from the psych ward, I'd gone to breakfast after a recovery meeting and come home much later than I'd said I would. I'm not the only one in the family who worries.

By afternoon, the spot on the bottom of my foot had disappeared along with the pain. Perhaps it was my shoes. I'd worn Newtons the day before, when it was painful, and Merrell Bare Access Arcs on this run. The next morning, our last in Ann Arbor, I ran five miles in the Newtons through neighborhoods and a small park. The new scenery and a few bursts of rain refreshed me. My left foot hurt a little, but not like before. I iced it and concluded that the increased miles and not the Newtons had caused the pain.

***

Back in Ohio on Saturday for our ten-mile fallback, a few of us fulls ran one mile in a light rain before joining the halfs who were doing nine. I again wondered who'd swapped my "not-a-morning-person" self for the new "before-dawn" version. Oh, the wonders of peer pressure. Neither Ed, an early riser, nor Mr. Dawg, who usually wants his breakfast at the crack of dawn, was awake at five when my alarm went off.

Our full group joined the halfs, waiting near the high school field house for Jeff, the Tall Guy, to call us to begin. The wind picked up and it began to rain sideways. While other groups headed into the weather, we clustered under the restroom overhang. Someone said, "We may be slow, but we're not stupid!"

Eventually we headed into the dark rain. Stephen, who had recovered nicely from his dizzy spells after a medication change, and his wife, Tereza, back from their run, came toward us wearing hats with clip-on headlamps. Stephen loaned me his headlamp since the trail was dark. Cold rain continued to pour. I worried I might chafe, but the Ohio State technical shirt Julie had given me for my birthday performed well.

Despite the pouring rain, we laughed about breast reduction surgery, bras, peeing your pants, and hypochondria. The miles flew. Ten miles had become a short run. In that downpour, I felt like a badass.

On the drive home, I called Ed from my car. After I'd left that morning, he'd awakened to thunder and lightning and worried about our group. He was relieved we'd had a fun, safe run. He was headed to a speech by a person who had escaped from a religious cult. I joked, "I've escaped into a running cult!"

***

When the pain in the bottoms of my feet returned, Janice, my therapist, who is also a yoga teacher, suggested it might be the new teal Newtons. After a few more painful runs in them, I bought a gently-used pair of the previous-model orange Newtons, on eBay after inspecting photos of the soles. On my first run in them, the increased comfort let me know I'd found my race-day shoes.

But my feet still hurt. When the pain began, a coach had suggested icing them, but I'm lazy. Now, I used two flexible ice packs, one on the sole and one on top, across the metatarsals. I even tried wearing my Brook Ravennas because they have more cushion. In those, my feet went numb, so I had no pain until after the run was over.

Pain brought nightmares. I woke in a cold sweat from a dream in which I stood on the sidelines while my friends ran the race. I tried to imagine carrying supplies and cheering for them at the finish. Injury had forced other friends to stop training or to drop to the half. At races, they smiled and cheered. I wasn't that mature. I distracted myself by bending my toes and pressing them on the floor. I did ankle circles and squeezed my toes together. It all hurt.

I frequently texted Julie to ask if she thought I had a stress fracture.

"Sharp pain?" she asked.

"No. Dull ache."

"That's good."

Stress fractures rarely show on x-rays for weeks, so I didn't go to the doctor. I continued icing and wearing the new (old model) Newtons and kept running.

***

A few weeks earlier, after our ten-mile run, Julie and I realized we both had football tickets for the Saturday we were scheduled to run twenty miles. Ohio State was playing the University of California, Berkeley, Ed's alma mater. Julie suggested we run Sunday, but I had signed up for the third annual Steps for Sarcoma 5k, the race that had been my first 5k back in 2010 and which my family planned to attend as a memorial to my niece.

Julie's eyes sparkled. "Let's do both!" We would run on Sunday before the race. Run the 5k. Then run the rest after. It was so crazy it might work. We recruited others for "The Great Twenty-Mile Adventure."

On Saturday, we watched the Ohio State Buckeyes beat the Berkeley Golden Bears fifty-two to thirty-four. That night, I did more than my usual pre-long-run tossing and turning in anticipation of the next morning's "adventure." Had I calculated the miles properly? Were the water stops and bathrooms in the right places? Would my friends like the course? Could I actually run twenty miles? It would be the furthest I'd ever run.

I intended to put coolers of water and bananas at Griggs Reservoir and Oxford Park, which we would pass more than once. Neither location has street lights. During my restless sleep, I'd dreamed that a man wearing a *ichigan hoodie had come up behind me, put a knife to my throat, and dragged me toward the Scioto River while I was setting out the coolers. The next morning, before dawn, when it was time to place them, I woke Ed and begged him to go along. He rolled over with his eyes closed. "You're really afraid?" When I told him about my nightmare, he pulled on clothes and went to the car. Back at the house, Ed kissed me and crawled back into bed.

It was still dark when Jennifer, Julie, and I left my sleeping husband for the neighborhood streets. The moon lit our way. At the intersection of Riverside Drive and Nottingham, we all jumped when the audible pedestrian crossing signal screeched. We crossed the wide, empty street to the park entrance.

Street lights illuminated this section of Griggs, but I still jumped at every noise. Fishermen with boats on trailers behind big pickups drove past slowly. This made me feel safer. If we encountered trouble, we could yell for them. Also, a police station sits on a hill at the south end of the park and police patrol regularly. As we jogged past the marina, the tree trunks and the road were dark, but the sky continued to brighten.

As usual, four miles in, I had to use the bathroom. We ran through tall, wet grass to the building on the hill. We couldn't figure out the light, so held the door open.

Near Fairfax, we crossed Riverside Drive into my favorite part of our neighborhood, a green, lush section with sycamores, maples, and large houses on big lots. As we approached tiny Oxford Park, I couldn't see the stashed cooler and became convinced someone had stolen it. Eventually I spotted it, down a slight incline, below street level. Julie and Jennifer laughed at me for being so paranoid.

We needed to be at the race by 7:45 a.m. to find my family and friends and the other MIT folks who would join us. I was certain we wouldn't make it, so we took a shortcut up the steep McCoy hill. My legs were strong and light with adrenaline. It had been forty-five degrees when we started and now was fifty—perfect running weather. As we crested the hill, race music filled the air. When I saw the inflatable arch in the distance, I sighed in relief. As usual, my worry was for naught.

At the park, we hugged my family, friends, and MIT runners Sue and LeDawn. The race didn't start on time, so Julie, Jennifer, and I ran around the park to stay warm. When the crowded race finally started, we took it slow. When the race doubled back and the leader blew past us, head down and sprinting, we cheered. How different I was from him. I was just happy to get through the miles.

When Jennifer, Julie, and I crossed the finish line together, a volunteer pulled me aside. Unlike last year when the race had given me an age group medal by mistake, this year I really had placed third in my age group. I called Ed. Like last year, he was again at the humanist brunch. I listened over the phone as he bragged about me to his friends.

My sister and I hugged and shed tears in memory of Jamey, her daughter. We took photos for Facebook, then Julie, Jennifer, Sue, LeDawn, and I continued the adventure by running back to our house, where Mr. Dawg barked until we came in. After a short break, we headed back to Oxford Park on our way to Griggs again.

This time when we crossed Riverside, at nearly ten o'clock, there was traffic. Jennifer didn't make it across with us and someone yelled, "No woman left behind!" while we waited.

Now the sun sparkled on the Scioto, turning it myriad shades of blue. The trees shone green and a slight breeze moved the leaves. Thirteen miles in, I felt tired, but not as much as I thought I would by this point. About a 10k to go. We cheered every mile. The temperature had risen to sixty degrees and I wished I'd remembered sunscreen.

The park teemed with people. The fishermen we'd seen earlier were now on the water, the skeletons of their trailers left behind. Two police officers drove by slowly, and one gave us a thumbs-up. Other runners waved. "Sixteen down. Four to go!" I yelled, eliciting another thumbs-up. Families had picnics with children. Couples walked hand in hand. Runners ran, bicyclists cycled, and people walked dogs. Gratitude filled me at being so fortunate to live near this beautiful sliver of green and blue.

My friends exclaimed over how pretty the course was, enjoying the shade and breeze along the river. Whenever a speedboat passed, we hoped to see men water-skiing, but had no luck. One of the police officers had nice dimples, so that was our only "hottie" sighting. No shirtless runners or cyclists. Perhaps all the hotties were at church.

The hill by the police station was difficult this time. My legs hurt and my sock rubbed my left little toe. I tried to ignore it, but the women insisted I stop to rearrange my sock.

Near the entrance, at the bottom of the big hill, I said something about walking, but Julie charged ahead and I followed. A few feet from the top, gasping, dizzy and lightheaded, I thought my heart would explode. Julie bent over, holding her knees.

We recovered for a minute, then crossed Riverside Drive when the audible pedestrian crossing signal told us to. Sue, who hadn't been with us to be startled by it in the quiet darkness earlier that morning, yelled, "Holy shit, that thing's loud!" and we all laughed.

The closer we got to our house, the stronger I felt, so much stronger than on the eighteen-mile run where I'd wanted to die the last three miles. Anticipating Julie's usual question, I told her I thought I could do another six. "Good for you," she said flatly. "You're in the zone." She wasn't. She'd taken a turbo caffeine gel before pounding up that hill. Her heart had skipped a beat and scared her. She was putting one foot in front of another, just trying to finish. I sent her some silent strength vibes from the glowing sensations that flooded me. I felt incredible! "You're pushing the pace," she snapped and pulled back. She was right. I'd flipped into hypomania. Adrenaline pulsed through me. Weren't we amazing? Everything sparkled.

But I'd miscalculated the mileage. Nobody wanted "extra credit," so we ran down into the ravine, then back to our house and past it a few houses, to get exactly twenty miles. My joy was palpable when Julie's watch beeped.

Morgan barked wildly at us from behind the kitchen window as we collapsed on the front porch to take off our shoes, drink water, and eat bananas. I yelled at him to stop, but he continued to howl. After Ed's brunch, he had gone to see the Richard Gere and Susan Sarandon film, *Arbitrage*, a thriller I didn't care to watch. Then he was canvassing for a presidential candidate. It took a few minutes of Morgan's barking before it occurred to me to let him out.

I gave the ladies confused directions about how to get to the restaurant we were going to next. Regardless, we arrived, ordered, and ate. I was high. I wanted to stay with these powerful women all day, but everyone had places to go. One by one, we left.

CHAPTER 24

Taper Madness

The day after "The Great Twenty-Mile Adventure," I had seven miles on the schedule. While were in *ichigan, Morgan had contracted kennel cough, essentially a doggie cold. He improved quickly with antibiotics and codeine, and the vet cleared him to run, but I didn't want to chance a recurrence. He barked at me through the kitchen window as I stood in the yard with my wrist in the air, trying to get my watch to auto-locate satellites. But I hadn't finished all seven miles before it was time to write with my ultramarathoning friend Wendy via Skype.

After Wendy and I finished, I took Mr. Dawg out to complete my seven. My legs were stiff. The back of my right knee and the fronts of both knees ached. These new pains spun my mind. A marathon was impossible.

Political signs dotted the yards. This was a presidential year and the nation was on edge. It didn't matter which party the signs supported, they annoyed me. I longed for the green simplicity of empty yards.

In the ravine, I had to drag Morgan out of the road as a man in a white van roared through. His radio blared and he was eating a slice of pizza. I yelled, "Twenty-five!" but he was long gone. When it was time for me to head home and go to therapy, I still didn't have seven. I searched for gratitude. It was sunny and the sky was deep blue. Some folks were still on the sofa.

The next day I woke from a dream in which a skunk had sprayed my whole family, including Morgan. It only took moments for me to decide I needed to run to shake off the dream and calm down. Ed called while we were running. We only talked for a minute, but this reminded me I was loved.

My knees were sore, but I let my body go slack and the pain evaporated. The ball and heel of my right foot hurt, but only mildly. Remembering our encounter with the white van the day before, I kept Morgan on a short leash. He wanted to sniff and pee, but I said, "Today is my run." Up the hill we went. At the top, I praised him.

***

I continued earning points toward my badass merit badge during midweek runs. After a run in a harsh headwind I thought might blow us over, I told the dog, "It's good practice in case it's windy on race day." He stuck his nose into the wind and squinted.

The next day, a friend mowing her lawn gave me a thumbs-up. The dog held his head high as we passed.

Then, a man about my age who I often see running said hello. In full brag mode, I called out, "Thirty days 'til the marathon." He stopped. "You're running the marathon?" I blushed and said, "That's my intention." He let out a whoop. A rush of positive sensations spread through my body. We high-fived and parted. Then I noticed men trimming trees a few yards away. I hoped they heard too.

Our running group's "mere" twelve-mile fallback should be easy, I thought. We full marathoners went out at 5:45 a.m. and ran 2.5 before our MIT group started. I was happy this was the last time we would have to get up early to start before the halfs. Eight miles in, my knee, legs, groin, and the bottoms of my feet ached. I was ready to be done. When I run with other people, I catch their rhythm and my cadence slows. I turned on my metronome for a few seconds to check my foot turnover, then switched it off so the beep didn't annoy the others. Tired and slouching, I did a few posture resets, then nearly herniated myself with a coughing fit. When I thought of next week's twenty-miler, I shook off the fear and returned my focus to this run. Keep your head where your feet are, I told myself.

At home, happy to be finished, I took a hot shower, then "hung off the stairs." This is my nickname for my favorite Egoscue e-cise, the "gravity drop." I placed the balls of my feet on the bottom step of our basement stairs, hung onto the handrail, and allowed gravity to stretch my body from head to toe. After that, I rolled my leg muscles with the stick.

***

The next day, despite how much slower my long runs had been, I placed third in my age group at Taking Strides for Kids 5k for a new personal record. Lots of kids and only a few older adults ran the Creekside course in downtown Gahanna. The first male came in at a sizzling 16:45. I received a hand-painted wooden bowl from the children of the Short Stop Youth Center, part of the Directions for Youth and Families program. Julie had volunteered, and we ate slices of pizza afterward.

Eight grueling miles followed that 5k PR. I'd worn the softer, higher-heeled Ravennas. It seemed my feet now preferred flatter shoes. If the marathon was anything like this, I would die. I didn't have the dog to talk to, and the *Three Non Joggers* humor I usually enjoyed sounded juvenile. I tried to convince myself that cheering fans, funny signs, and water stops would distract me on marathon day, but didn't believe it. I chanted, "This is the mile you came to run," and "Bring the body and the mind will follow." Difficult days trained the mind as much as the body.

Two days later the dog and I PR'd a six-mile course in the pouring rain. Instead of listening to *Three Non Joggers*, I focused on form, keeping my body upright and knees bent. I picked up my feet and kicked them behind me with no knee pain. Because of the weather, only the lady with the Border Collie was out. Even the trash men wore slickers. We were earlier than normal, so people headed to work and dropping kids at school filled the streets we usually found empty. I hopped into the grass several times to avoid cars during the first two miles, before traffic thinned. At a construction site, I snuck into the porta potty. Mr. Dawg whined outside, but there wasn't room for us both. A few miles later, the Chihuahuas went nuts in their bay window. Their mom waved as Morgan peed on the big shrub at the corner of their property. I felt ready for Saturday and our second twenty-miler.

That week, at another Good Form Running Clinic, this time at Fleet Feet, Jeff, the Tall Guy, talked about core and taught A, B, and C drills. In addition, he suggested I do Russian twists, disc-weight arm exercises, and tilts. Jeff noticed that I look down when I run and recommended that I focus on posture all day long. He didn't video me as I had hoped, but when he pointed to the bottoms of my "new" Newtons and the wear showed I was still heel-striking, I groaned. On my next run, I tried to keep my body upright. I tilted my pelvis, made sure my shoulders were back, and focused on a tree in the distance instead of the ground.

***

The final Saturday in September, our MIT schedule showed twenty-two miles. Julie, Jennifer, LeDawn, and I intended to cut it to twenty, but somewhere between Henderson and North Broadway, nine miles in, we caught stadium fever and decided to run it all. Twenty-two miles! Two years before, I'd barely jogged for sixty seconds down in the ravine while carrying a kitchen timer.

I'd run the first five and a half miles with the faster halfs and, by the time I took my first potty break at the Worthington Hills gazebo, I was in pain. After another potty break at the Park of Roses, a wave of hopelessness passed through me and "No way" began an involuntary mantra in my head. I brushed it aside. If I wanted to stay with my friends, I had to keep going. It wasn't that far to the next water stop. I picked up my feet.

Faster runners came back up the trail toward us. The stadium, fondly referred to by locals as "the Shoe" for its horseshoe shape, was open and Jeff, the Tall Guy, was taking photos. That fueled me from Dodridge to Schottenstein Arena.

Food also helped. Julie's boyfriend Reg had left bananas at the Como water stop and Jennifer had left bananas by the trailhead near Thomas Worthington High School. I'd packed peanut butter crackers. At the corner of Lane Avenue and Olentangy River Road, Fred Girscht, a multiple-organ-transplant survivor and fellow member of MIT, offered peanut butter and jelly sandwiches. The sweet and salty combination melted in my mouth. MITers know how to take care of each other.

When Julie took us under the Lane Avenue bridge, I went a little nuts, convinced we would get lost. She smirked, then smiled. "I've done this before." I apologized and followed. I hit another porta potty by Woody Hayes Drive.

But Jeff wasn't at the Shoe when we arrived. A kindly freshman orientation usher welcomed us onto the field and took photos of us doing O-H-I-O. Jennifer texted the photo to Jeff, "Where's the love for our pace group?" Jeff texted back, explaining he'd chosen to make sure we had hydration instead. Earlier in the season, we had run out of water, so Jennifer texted back, "Hydration is important." The adult part of me knew Jeff made the right choice, but I snarked and complained like a pissy three-year-old as we ran around the outside of the Shoe. I was afraid our photos wouldn't wind up on the MIT Facebook page. Everyone else had let it go.

When we left the Shoe, pain forced both Jennifer and LeDawn to walk. Julie said we had peaked there. Having recovered from my tantrum, I said I'd peaked at the peanut butter and jelly sandwich.

To combat my lagging spirits, I mentally broke the next section into parts: Stadium to Ackerman Road to the driveway of the wetlands to the little building to the bridge to the water stop at Como. Julie said she was doing something similar.

At the Como water stop, a woman runner we didn't recognize was holding our cached bag of bananas. As I sped toward her, she set them down and walked away. I handed the bag to Julie who doled out the precious fruit to each of us. "Good thing she didn't mess with our bananas!" Julie said. We agreed. We were in no mood to not have bananas.

Through the neighborhood north of North Broadway, Julie looked wary. She had read an article about children being attacked by pit bulls. I shared the encounters Mr. Dawg and I had had with loose dogs. We both heard dog noises, but there were no dogs.

Julie asked if it was harder to run with just Morgan or with people. I said it's just different. Sometimes it's harder with people because I don't keep my own pace. But the dog doesn't talk, so the group is more entertaining.

I needed another pee break at the Park of Roses. In my usual hypochondriacal fashion, I worried I might have a urinary tract infection. The next day, I would be fine.

On the secluded, two-mile stretch from Henderson Road to Antrim Lake, I watched for and named the landmarks: bench, tree, chain-link fence. "We're playing mind games," I said. Delirious, but breathing fine, Julie asked, "Can I play too?" I'd meant the landmarks game and her face sagged when I said, "We're already playing them." She laughed. "I'm like a three-year-old. Tell me a story." I declined. I might be a writer but can't make up stories on a run.

Instead of stories, I mentioned the brilliant red poison ivy leaves. "But we won't touch it," I joked. She didn't laugh. She was beyond laughter. Mentally, I felt solid. The landmark game and entertaining Julie occupied me. By contrast, Julie seemed physically strong, while my legs were heavy. I tried to refocus on form, but two steps of good form gave way to twenty of heel-striking. I also tried to focus ahead. I told Julie about y'chi from ChiRunning, where you focus your eyes on a faraway object and let it pull you toward it. "Not now," she said. We trudged onward. These difficult miles were the ones we had come to run.

Back at Antrim, Jeff was dumping the extra water. Julie and I wondered if he was angry that we'd made a big deal out of his not being at the Shoe. But twenty miles into a twenty-two-miler was not the time to figure that out.

LeDawn, Jennifer, and four others were well behind Julie and me now. Julie phoned Jennifer, who said not to wait. She and LeDawn were in too much pain to catch us. We alerted Jeff and, when Jennifer and LeDawn arrived at Antrim, Jeff drove them back to the high school.

Between Antrim and Route 161, Julie repeatedly asked me to slow down. The closer to the finish, the faster I go.

At the last water station, I asked if we were stopping. Julie shook her head, "I might not start again." At the stop sign, neither of us had twenty-two miles on our watches. "Around the lot!" I commanded. That warm "almost done" glow, a blend of exquisite pain and exhilarating joy, filled my body.

Jennifer and LeDawn cheered while Jeff slammed tables and water jugs. I was certain he was angry but would learn later that he was trying to avoid being stung by the bees drawn to the Gatorade.

Jennifer yelled, "Last but not least!" since we were last of the running group to finish. I yelled, "We may be slow, but we're not stupid!" referring to the day our group had taken shelter from a thunderstorm while the faster pace groups ran straight into it. Then Julie looked at her watch and yelled, "Twenty-two!"

Standing around afterward, I felt proud, but so exhausted. I worried about Jennifer and LeDawn but had no energy for conversation. We crawled into our cars and left. Later, Jeff apologized to Jennifer for not being at the Shoe and used our O-H-I-O photo as the cover of a video he posted about the twenty-two-mile run.

The next day my hunger was enormous and my ankle painful to put weight on. Moving it helped. Still, my body amazed me. We'd been out there almost six hours.

When we'd been running the parking lot to get our final mileage, Julie had asked, "How many more miles could you run?" I didn't hesitate. "Four point two." That's all I needed to know.

***

After our twenty-two-mile run, I didn't run for three days. This was my longest break since I'd begun to train for the full. When I woke that third morning, still burned out, my mind told me three miles was impossible. It said I'd lost all my fitness and running would be horrible. I leashed up the dog anyway, focused on picking up my feet and knees, my body a blob of ache.

That evening, we ran after dark at the MIT midweek six-mile run. My knee, hip, and ankle hurt, and I had to push to keep up. My headlamp was dim, and when Julie whispered, "There's something over there," we started sprinting. It turned out to be another runner. Later, I thought the sign for the footbridge was a person and nearly knocked Sue down.

A few days later, when I was still in bed, heavy with muscle aches and lethargy, a loud *BOOM!* cracked against the bedroom window. A hawk with a squirrel still in its talons sat on the ground, shaken, having flown into the window. The squirrel scurried off unharmed, while the hawk shook itself, then flew away. I took that as my sign to shake out my still painful legs. On our run, the Chihuahuas barked at Morgan and bounced merrily in their bay window. The woman who always wears a dress walked with her keeshond on a leash and her untethered cat following behind. Mr. Dawg and I greeted them all, as I continued to check my form. In the marathon, I would need to check every mile and relax. And I would need to not worry about my friends. We would all run our own races.

Saturday brought the kind of sparkling fall weather I love, cold but sunny, with autumn leaves shining against a bright blue sky. Both MIT groups, halfs and fulls, ran twelve together. As was typical, I feared getting lost. I tried to keep up while periodically checking my cadence with my metronome but couldn't. I gave up and hung back with Mike Marshall. We both grew up in the country and talk of livestock and crops made the miles fly. When the group turned, I had warmed up enough to stay with them.

At home, I put my aching left foot in a bucket of ice water and stifled a scream. I lasted five minutes. I'd run too hard and vowed not to go out so fast during the marathon. I switched to my right and when it was done, I stuck my left foot back in the ice and tolerated it better. I was so ready for that hot shower!

I took two days off to let my foot return to normal, but it was still sore when I went for a diagnostic run. A metatarsal in my right foot had been sore and swollen since Saturday's twelve-mile run. I feared the dreaded stress fracture. I had rested instead of doing the five-mile run, but when I tried our six-mile run, my foot ached after two miles. I remembered Julie's question. No, the pain was not sharp.

I thought about calling Dr. Bright, the medical director for the Columbus Marathon, but decided against it. He might tell me I couldn't run the marathon, and I couldn't accept that. I needed to rest. But if I rested until the race, I feared I'd be so out of shape I wouldn't be able to finish or would be too slow to meet the time limit. I didn't know what else to do, so I iced it again. Surely I had a stress fracture. Maybe the pain was from my "new" orange version of Newtons. No. They were more comfortable. I did not know.

I was in the throes of "taper madness." Without the long runs to burn off anxiety, my mind spun trying to fix the problem. Random aches and pains surfaced, adding to the confusion.

By the next day, the swelling had gone down enough to run with the dog. My foot didn't hurt while I ran, but my legs grew heavy after four miles. The last two were so slow that, as in our beginning days of running, Morgan barely had to trot to keep up. I stopped to pee at the construction site porta potty, but still peed my pants. I wasn't sure what I'd do on race day.

After the run, my foot ached. Ice. Ibuprofen. Compression. Elevation. That was the plan. I would run this marathon. When it was over, I might get the foot checked. Maybe.

***

A week before the marathon, Ed and I traveled to Portland, Oregon, for him to attend a conference and then to Seattle to again visit his older son, Ken. The first morning in Portland, I was unhappy with our small hotel room, not impressed with what little I'd seen of the city, and just tired. As always, I was afraid to run because I thought I would get lost. I went anyway. Runners, cyclists, and two homeless men sharing a joint entertained me on the path along the Willamette River. I ran under the smaller bridges, but not the path over the river, beneath the massive, steel suspension bridge. I have my limits.

I ran on a boardwalk at the edge of the river, but when the path snaked under another huge bridge, I turned around. A flight of Canada geese took off in formation from the silver surface of the river and brightened my mood. Back at the hotel, I smiled at the sweaty clothes hanging over the television and lamps. This made me a real runner. I'd navigated the city on foot. That made me a real runner. My body, except for my foot, felt great. I iced it and wore support hose all day. That too, made me a real runner.

A few days before, Ed had been honored with the House of Hope Award for his work as Chief Financial Officer of the long-term residential treatment facility. We'd planned this trip before he knew about the award, but Ed had made reservations at Portland City Grill and we intended to celebrate.

Unfortunately, when I tried to board the express elevator to the restaurant on the thirtieth floor, my throat closed, my breath grew shallow, and my vision blurred. Certain I would pass out, I convinced Ed to take two elevators instead. At dinner, I concentrated on the twinkling city lights visible from our window table and the succulent meal. Afterward, I forced myself to ride the express elevator down.

The next morning, I ran the opposite direction, toward Washington Park. A glimpse out our fifteenth-floor hotel room window toward the huge hill might have clued me in to the terrain, but I'd just been worried about crossing the freeway. Right before the park stood a buckeye tree. I took a photo of the large pile of "worthless nuts" lying at the base of the tree and picked up two for luck, one for me and one for my sister Amy, who is also an Ohio State alumna.

I took photos in the International Rose Test Garden and the Portland Japanese Garden. Then I turned up Kingston, trying to focus on form, but the gentle uphill switchbacks proved challenging. I walked the steepest hills up and up and up. At the zoo, I lost my bearings and panicked. I forced myself to just keep breathing until I found the turnaround at Hoyt Arboretum. My quads burned as I let my feet roll up behind me, and I barreled back down. A short rain shower refreshed me. The little store at the Rose Garden was now open, so I bought a refrigerator magnet and sampled their rose tea. Then I ran past the hotel to Salmon Springs, around the fountain and back to the hotel. After my shower, I iced my foot and cheered myself. I had run those hills, navigated another strange city, and kept myself moving.

The next day, we took Amtrak to rainy Seattle, where Ken met us at the station. Earlier in the year, when we'd been there, I'd run the eastern route around Lake Union. This time I ran five miles around the west side to the Aurora Bridge. I focused on keeping my head up, my pelvis tilted, and my feet quick. I only used the metronome once, but my cadence was good. My quads still hurt from the Portland hills.

The street view had made the trail beneath the Aurora Bridge look secluded, so I'd left the hotel with some trepidation. The area turned out to be well-traveled. Construction workers carried a door past a man using a jackhammer, so I covered my ears. A man getting a claw hammer out of his car said hello. Several runners waved. Bearded men in tight jeans and flannel shirts greeted me as they walked their dogs. Four young men, all carrying sandwich bags, stepped aside politely for me. I said, "I'm slow. If I hit you, it won't leave a dent." They laughed. I took more photos. As usual, I had been afraid, but wound up having fun. Afterward, I iced my foot.

***

Back in Columbus, excited and terrified at the prospect of Sunday's marathon, I stuck to the training schedule. The dog and I ran three miles Wednesday in unseasonably warm sun, while gusts of wind blew crisp leaves across the ground. Early in the run, thoughts of race day and how much it might hurt made my chest tighten with fear. Articles about race strategy came to mind, fueling the panic. I run based on feel and just wanted to finish. I turned my attention to my strong arms and legs and the anxiety passed.

Halfway through our run, Morgan and I saw Jim, our mail carrier. "Any marathon advice?" I asked. He gave Morgan the usual biscuit then, stern-faced, he pointed a finger near my nose and said, "Have fun!"

For the rest of the run, I focused on my surroundings, allowing signs for politicians I didn't appreciate to slide over me despite my upset stomach. The second 2012 presidential debate had been the night before. I pushed away images of my candidate conceding to the candidate I deplored. "Keep your mind where your feet are,"

I reminded myself. The election wasn't for thirteen days. The marathon was in four. By this time Sunday, the race would be over.

After this run, my ankle didn't hurt, but I iced it as a precaution.

Friday, I took the dog for two miles. The point, I explained to Mr. Dawg, was to remember that I know how to run without exerting myself too close to the race. I couldn't believe the race was so soon. I tried to remember the training. Well, not the eighteen-miler that nearly killed me, but the twenty-miler when we ran a 5k in the middle and the twenty-two miler to Ohio Stadium when Fred gave us sandwiches. I also tried to forget the twelve-miler when I thought I had a stress fracture and the days of foot pain following our trip to Ann Arbor.

I turned my attention to the smooth blonde back of Mr. Dawg, trotting easily beside me. I waved at the neighbor whose Golden Retriever and Irish setter dragged him down the street. The Chihuahuas barked and spun gleefully in their bay window. We dodged men working with huge collapsible pipes and pumps down in the ravine. Periodically, I reset my form—head up, quick foot turnover, feet light and easy, small steps—and reset my posture when Morgan stopped to pee.

As I entered the run in my log, I thought, "Next time I write here, I will have run a marathon!"

CHAPTER 25

———————

Earning My Sticker

Friday night, before the marathon, at the expo, I apologized to the volunteer when I dropped my full marathon bib. I couldn't steady my hands. My grip left fingerprints on the race T-shirt.

Anxiety and awkwardness rendered me nearly speechless when I met the handful of Dead Runners who had come from out of town to run the race. The others, reconnecting after only talking online for long periods of time, hugged and chatted. I talked to Carl and Lynn, then wandered away. Seeing some MIT friends calmed me a little. One of them pointed to a pink hat that read, "WTF!" on the front and "Where's the Finish?" on the back. Breaking the "nothing new on race day" rule, I bought it.

After the expo, when our pace group met to carb-load, nervous laughter filled our conversation. Sadly, since our twenty-two-mile run, LeDawn had been diagnosed with a fracture; however, she joined us for dinner, and we planned meeting spots.

Saturday morning, I met the Deads at Antrim Lake for a short walk, where the talk turned to race goals. Carl hoped to break four hours. I hoped to finish upright, preferably before dark.

Saturday afternoon, Ed and I trekked to the thrift store for throwaway clothes. I bought a black velvet hoodie with a rhinestone zipper pull I couldn't imagine throwing away. Then we went to some friends' house to watch Ohio State beat Purdue. Eventually, we went home so I could try to sleep.

***

We were late. I forgot my running shoes. My shoe laces came untied and I tripped and fell into a Gatorade table. I forgot to bring electrolyte gels or food, and no one would give me any. The gels I brought had caffeine, and I had repeated panic attacks. I couldn't find Julie, Jennifer, Sue, or anyone I'd hoped to run with. I wandered off the course. Once I found my way back, they had torn down the finish line, so my time didn't count and I didn't get a medal. I never found Ed or Amy or anyone else who was cheering for me. I missed the turn to the stadium, and they disqualified me for cutting the course. I had diarrhea. They altered the course at the last minute and we had to run down the highway through the I-70/I-71 split in full traffic. I was nearly plowed down by a semi whose driver refused to stop for the officer directing traffic. A small child spat on me. A dog bit me near mile seventeen and I had to go to the First Aid tent for stitches. It was hot and they ran out of water. It was cold and my fingers and feet went numb. I tripped on the timing mat at the finish and broke my nose. My doctor called early race morning to tell me I had a mysterious illness that would kill me if I ran. We had a flat tire on the way to the race and, by the time I arrived, the race was over. Ed had a heart attack waiting for me in the cold. I didn't hear my phone ring, so I ran the whole race while he lay dying. A sniper fired shots near mile eighteen and wasn't captured until he killed several spectators. I came in last. Then, I woke up.

***

The morning of the 2012 Columbus Marathon dawned crisp at forty degrees with lifting fog. I woke at four thirty. In the bathroom, I read motivational passages from the *Non-Runner's Marathon Trainer* about creative visualization, mantras, and flow states. I thought of Ryan Hall's admonition, "Run the mile you're in."

Morgan snuffled my lips then rubbed himself against my knees, begging for me to scratch him. I set the book down and obeyed. Once he was satisfied, I dressed in the gear I'd laid out the night before: pink WTF hat I'd bought at the expo, a blue tank top with a pink MIT logo, black capris, pink sport socks, and bright orange Newton shoes.

Ed dropped me at the Hyatt for the MIT pre-race gathering. In our throwaway clothes, oversized, mismatched, sweatshirts, pants, and hoodies layered over running gear, we looked homeless. Jimmy demonstrated his "breakaway" pajama pants, showing how quickly he could drop them. I proudly wore the fifty-two-cent black velvet hoodie and throwaway gloves. For arm warmers, Sue had cut the toes off a pair of black tube socks bearing the "CAT" logo of Caterpillar heavy machinery company. We snacked, giggled, stretched, and took photos to burn off nervous energy until Jeff, the Tall Guy, yelled, "Bags to the truck!" We did as instructed, then posed as Jeff took the group photo. My arms and legs tingled with excitement and fear.

Our running group of nearly a thousand people created a small parade as we headed down High Street. Official race photographers captured a group of us shivering. We stopped at the porta potties, then headed to Corral F: "Fun and Fabulous." Ed had been reading on the stairs of a heated underground parking garage until I called. He had a cold and was trying not to catch pneumonia. He wound his way to us, and I hugged and kissed him.

Each time the statehouse cannon fired, I jumped, craning my neck to see the tops of the fireworks being set off at Broad and Third, the actual start line. This was before the Boston bombing, so we knew it was just the cannon, but those blasts, combined with standing smushed together in the corral, made me lightheaded. Shivering, I thought I might throw up. When our corral moved, I kissed Ed goodbye, then waved as he took photos from atop the base of a street lamp. I fell silent but listened as the others nervously chatted.

As we walked, I calmed my nerves by rehearsing my race day affirmation, "Run easy. Run strong." How far I'd come. In two and a half years, I'd gone from running for sixty seconds, down in the hidden neighborhood ravine, to toeing the line of my first full marathon in a crowd of eighteen thousand runners and who knows how many spectators. Close quarters still made me uncomfortable, so I focused on slow breathing. Phantom aches floated through my body, and worry spun my mind.

Just before we crossed the start, Jennifer cried, "My watch timed out!" We stepped aside to let others pass while Jennifer waved her arm in the air. "Got it!" she yelled. One by one, we crossed and started our individual watches.

Now came true panic. This was really it! It was a huge relief to no longer be in the crush of the corrals, but wow. Again, I grew lightheaded. "Stay in this mile," I thought. Sue and several others had found David, LeDawn's husband, and went to run the half with him. The rest of us ran together for the first three miles. Stephen joined us.

Julie and I had ditched our hoodies and gloves before the start. We thought we would warm up quickly now that we were running. It was warm between buildings, but, at each intersection, the cold October wind blew along the cross-street. Even rubbing my bare arms didn't help. My teeth chattered and goosebumps rose on my arms and legs. Jimmy joked about picking up the throwaway gloves that littered the ground. "I'd wear a used pair," I said. Jimmy picked them up. He picked up pairs for Julie and Jennifer too, then took a video of us doing jazz hands in our thrown-away throwaway gloves.

We were still downtown when I spotted someone riding a bicycle in a yellow chicken costume. That chicken was tall! Jeff, "the Tall Guy," usually dressed in a Bigfoot costume. But as the chicken caught and passed us, Jeff's grinning face peeked out of the costume's beak. He pointed a camera and we hammed.

Before Bexley, Stephen, Jimmy, and Robert left Julie, Jennifer, and me behind. Near mile three, we went under the railroad bridge, where the man in the kilt again played bagpipes. I swallowed tears.

I'd been sipping water and thought the bathroom business was going fine, but as we ran through Bexley, I felt the urge to pee. I told Julie and Jennifer I would need to stop. I reminded them of the pact we had to each run our own race. I did not expect them to wait.

Cheering fans and trees in fall foliage peppered the streets near Jeffrey Mansion and the Governor's Mansion. When we arrived at the porta potty between miles four and five, I needed to stop, but there was a line. During the previous mile, I had warned them I would need to stop and told them to go ahead. Now they hesitated but went on. I figured that was the last time I'd see them before the finish.

Once I was inside, my mind attacked.

"Who do you think you are?" said the familiar critic.

Grotesque images arose. The waxy feel of Dad's skin as he lay dead in the hospice house. Mom struggling as a nurse tried to remove her ventilator tube. The look on Jamey's boyfriend's face as he carried my niece's dead body down their apartment stairs.

Crouched over the toilet seat, I shook my head, trying to clear the images from my mind.

Yes, I was alone now and these loved ones were gone. But I carried their memories inside me. I had trained for this race. They would want me to do my best to finish.

A knock on the plastic door reminded me about the line of runners waiting. I finished my task.

Before I opened the door, I whispered, "I'm a runner!" Then I pulled up my panties and stepped out.

As my feet touched the grass, the porta potty wobbled. The man next in line steadied me. "That was close," he said. We both laughed. He had no idea.

***

Then, I made my first mistake. I tried to catch Julie and Jennifer. I figured I was five minutes behind. Determined, I focused on my form and settled into my stride, pushing through Bexley onto Main, back toward downtown. It was misty and beautiful.

My feet grew tired and my heart lonely, but knowing Jennifer and Julie were ahead pulled me on. This was my fastest part of the race. My body had warmed up, and I ditched the secondhand gloves. Conserving energy, I paid no attention to race signs and didn't high-five anyone. When I took the little turn in Old Towne East through a neighborhood with lots of spectators, I pulled their energy into me. As I crossed the bridge over I-71, I remembered balking at the towering freeway in Seattle. Not today.

In German Village, a man sitting at an outdoor table smiled as I ran past Katzinger's Deli. I forgot to conserve energy and asked if he had a salami on rye for me. "With mustard or without?" he replied and held out his half-eaten sandwich. In Schiller Park, I gave the overhead race photographers my best smile. I planned to buy all the photos.

Just beyond the photographer's arch, I spotted Julie and Jennifer. "Hey coaches!" I yelled, but they didn't hear. I sped up and yelled again. They still didn't hear. I cupped my hands around my mouth and screamed, "MIT Coaches!" Julie looked back, saw me, then grinned and waved. Jennifer saw me and beamed too. "Best moment ever!" Jennifer said when I caught them. Julie said they had been wondering about me for miles. Jennifer said, "You must have run fast!" I shrugged, trying to act nonchalant. "I relaxed and leaned," I said, but inside I was roaring with glee. A woman dressed as a cow passed us. Another runner declared her "udderly spectacular."

Ahead, Stephen was leaning on a tree, stretching. His daughters and his son-in-law were on bicycles on the course. He'd had a rough week but hoped to finish the full. He was listening to meditation podcasts to stay in the moment. His wife, a stronger, faster runner, had taken off earlier.

From German Village to Nationwide Boulevard, the halfway point, is about two and a half miles. It's a long, slow climb, with little scenery except the Ohio Statehouse and Columbus Commons. We saw Juli (no "e"), a member of our pace group, near the I-70 overpass, cheering and taking photos. Back at the Statehouse, I spotted the street lamp Ed had stood on earlier that morning to take our photo. Jennifer said, "Were we just here several hours ago?" Julie looked at her watch. "Two hours and forty-nine minutes ago."

A black pile of cloth on the ground caught my eye. Printed in white were the letters "CAT." Sue's arm warmers! This reminder of her warmed me. I hoped she'd achieved her half marathon PR.

Mile eleven, the "Angel Mile," is dedicated to the patients of Nationwide Children's Hospital who did not survive their illnesses. We grew quiet, looking at banner photos of the young darlings no longer on the planet. I thought of Jamey. She'd been an adult, but I wanted to remember her as that little blonde tyke I'd taken shopping.

Near mile twelve, the MIT cheer squad, including my writing friend Jacqui and her husband George, called to us. I fought back tears every time someone cheered.

As we neared the half turnoff, people yelled, "You're almost there!" We pointed to our blue marathon bibs and yelled back, "NOT!" The half marathon bibs were orange. We felt pretty badass when we crested the hill by the Nationwide tower.

In the middle of High Street, the injured LeDawn appeared before us like a gift. When she saw us, she held up the ziplock bags of supplies we'd given her at the hotel. Julie opened her arms and squealed. Jennifer laughed, and I choked back more tears. Thanking her profusely, I took my bag and crossed Nationwide Boulevard. Race marshals yelled and motioned the halfs to veer left to their finish and for us fulls to continue up High Street.

"We missed our turn," Jennifer said. Only another half marathon to go.

**

On the four-and-a-half-mile High Street stretch through the Short North and Ohio State, I suggested stopping at Jeni's Ice Cream. Julie said she planned to go post-race. Jennifer wanted Betty's. I ate another gel.

In front of Ohio Union, a band played "It's Raining Men." Race marshals danced in the street on the right as cute college guys staffed a water stop on the left. "It really is raining men!" Jennifer said.

I'd broken up the long, straight stretch of High Street from German Village to Lane Avenue in my mind, the same way I had the seemingly endless sections of the Olentangy Trail, but my legs ached from those fast miles when I'd chased Jennifer and Julie. It relieved me to have caught them, but my body paid for it. Ohio Stadium lay ahead. I pushed to make it there.

Four hours into the day, many entertainers were tearing down. One musician grumbled, "This is a race, not a stroll," as we passed. "I'd like to see him run for six hours straight!" I grumbled.

Shortly after we turned from High Street to Lane Avenue, Jennifer fell behind. Julie slowed and asked if she was okay. I'm ashamed I didn't ask. I'd switched into survival mode. When Julie began to run again, I mentally Velcroed myself to her.

The Lane Avenue bridge came into view. I nudged Julie, then remembered the course map. It wasn't a straight shot down Lane. We had to cross the Olentangy, run to Fyfe Road, then turn back to Ohio Stadium. My body sagged, and I shuffled until I spotted Sarah, the full marathoner from the year before who had so inspired me with her blue "full" medal. She and Richard, another runner friend, held signs. "Got Runs?" and "26.2 is Sexy." I tried to clap, but only managed a limp wave.

It felt as if I'd been running forever. I brought my attention to my left foot as it hit the ground, lifted, then hit the ground again. My body swayed. In the race photos I would see later, I'm hunched like an old lady.

Ohio Stadium loomed, gray and enormous. We ran into the wind tunnel it created, followed the race flags to the steep ramp, and flew down. Julie recorded our entrance on her camera phone. I waved at my friend Jenny, who stood on the edge of the bleachers. Amy took video. Ed held out half a peanut butter and jelly sandwich. I grasped it in one hand and hugged him with the other. "I love you," I whispered in his ear.

When I turned back, Julie was gone. I raced to catch her as she plowed up the exit ramp to meet her family. They took a quick O-H-I-O photograph while I nibbled at the sandwich. I threw the rest in the trash and we were off again.

As we left the stadium, Julie said, "Single digits!" That didn't sound right, but math was, once again, beyond me. I looked back at the stadium getting smaller behind us and saw Jennifer. A pang of guilt shot through me at having left her. Julie and I waved, and Jennifer gave us a thumbs-up.

We saw Juli (no "e") again just past the stadium. The sign she held now read, "When the going gets tough, 'Punch it, Jake!'" referring to the motto we'd adopted from the father and his young son our running group had encountered that season. More tears to push away.

At Woody Hayes and Fyfe, a group of Columbus State students blocked the road. "Which way?" I yelled and a young woman pointed into the crowd. Grumpy at them for not taking the race seriously, I didn't recognize it as a water stop. This felt ominous. Plus, they wore matching navy-blue sweats like a sports team. I didn't think Columbus State had a sport team. I shook off the disorientation but became confused again as we headed into Ohio State's "west campus." I'd imagined us running down Kenny to Kinnear, but arrows pointed toward the office buildings near Fred Beekman park.

Post-stadium letdown hit. It had been great to see Juli with her "Punch It, Jake!" sign, but now we were in a no-man's-land of empty parking lots. Julie sensed my dismay and talked about people we hoped to see. I was so tired I didn't care. Those miles I'd run catching Julie and Jennifer continued to wear on me. I lost my form, my thoughts became scattered, and I kept zoning out. Julie might have enjoyed conversation, but I'm not much of a talker on a good day, and especially not at mile nineteen. Listening to *Three Non Joggers* might have helped, but I didn't think of it.

While I dragged, Julie bloomed. "Nita Sweeney! I think we can do this in 6:15." She hoped for a marathon PR in this, her second full. I was unsure how she'd come up with that number. She'd asked me to add two numbers. I told her they totaled ninety-eight. I'm not sure what the numbers were.

Once we were on Kinnear, I looked for my friend Marshall and my neighbor Luke, but the only person at the North Star intersection was a teenage boy in a black T-shirt carrying a notebook. I wondered how he could carry a notebook while racing. Eventually, I realized he was just going for a walk.

Spectators cheered in front of houses on Waltham in Upper Arlington. At mile twenty, after an announcer called our names, my friend Maureen appeared in the street, arms wide, unmistakable with her white hair and purple coat. I hugged her and her friend David. In a race, you hug everyone. Also on Waltham, we spotted another friend, Jim, walking. I hugged him. "See you at the finish," I said, trying to cheer him. "I'm a mental basket case," he said. I understood. If I hadn't been afraid of losing Julie, I too would have been walking.

A few minutes later, Julie asked where we were on the course. I'd driven the course on Friday to memorize it. I told her the next turn, but she couldn't visualize it. We came up behind someone in the official race shirt which had the course map on the back. I pointed and explained. Julie pointed, too, but accidentally poked the guy in the back. We apologized, but he gave us a dirty look. A moment later, Luke called to us. I hugged Luke, Dawn, and their darling red-haired daughters Tessa and Sienna, and thanked them for staying out there so long. Luke gave me his stoic smile. Later, Luke emailed me a photo he'd captured of Julie pointing at the back of that guy's shirt.

Next, I spotted a young man in a Mylar blanket lying in a yard. He looked so peaceful. Thinking he'd finished the race, I called, "Nice blanket!" He gave me a feeble thumbs-up. Julie whispered, "Nita! He's in the medic tent!" I yelled back, "Hope you're all right." Just another clue that by mile twenty my brain wasn't functioning. I was just going from point to point on the map in my head.

At Cambridge Road, Julie asked, "Are we on the end of that little bump-out on the left yet?" Then, "Do we have to go back north again?" I tried to explain but mumbled something incomprehensible. She abandoned her questions. I kept tripping on potholes, bumping into her, and apologizing. My gait was a shuffle.

The blocks on King crawled. At North Star, Julie asked, "Is this Grandview?" When I said "No," she seemed sad, but told me, "I feel like my old race Julie." Her first marathon had been brutally hot. Dehydration and pain had made her look half-dead in the photos. Today she smiled for every camera. While I was happy for her, I had no smiles left. I'd succumbed to "gut it out Nita" mode, plodding the pavement.

Julie's questions finally made sense when we spotted her partner Reg and her parents near Grandview and King. She hadn't told me she was watching for them. During the two-minute break while she grabbed a snack, I stared blankly up the road. I should have been stretching or eating the peanut butter and jelly sandwich I'd ditched at the stadium.

Long before I was ready, Julie began to run again. I followed. As we crossed Fifth Avenue in front of the Indian restaurant, I envied the two large men coming out with presumably full stomachs. On Grandview Avenue, after we crossed Third, an elderly man in an old Buick Century glided toward us in our lane. Traffic should be on the other side of the street. Deluded, I pushed Julie toward the car. She pushed back. Before we collided, I recognized my insanity and pulled her away. It didn't matter if the guy was in the wrong lane. We didn't need to become hood ornaments. A race marshal shrugged and shook her head.

In front of Jeni's Ice Cream, a pregnant woman and a tall man jogged toward us. It took several moments for me to recognize my friends Chris and Heather, the Turkey Trot and Rescue Run friends. Heather, nine months pregnant and, unbeknownst to me, scheduled to be induced the next morning, hugged me. Chris took a photo and I waved to Heather's parents, who were sitting in lawn chairs watching the race. Then Maureen and David appeared again. I hugged them, then noticed Julie pulling away. I caught her as we turned onto First.

At mile twenty-three, on the long hill down First Avenue, a tall, thin walker talking nonstop grated on my frayed nerves. "This is my fifty-third at this distance," he said, and told us we looked good. I wanted to smack him. Feeling weak, old, tired, and on the verge of tears, I wanted it over. It seemed impossible we only had a 5k to go. Math again. It might as well have been 100k. We passed the tall walker and his voice thankfully faded into the distance. At the bottom of the hill lay Northwest Boulevard.

Next came the incline at Edgehill. Anyone who tells you Columbus is flat has never run Upper Arlington and Grandview. They are gentle, rolling hills, but hills nonetheless.

Halfway up, my pounding heart made my breath turn shallow. My insides shook.

"I don't feel well," I muttered.

Julie didn't respond, perhaps chalking it up to the fact I was running uphill over twenty-three miles into my first marathon.

But soon, dizzy and lightheaded, I had to squint to see her. An aura formed on each side of my eyes and my vision blurred. I stumbled and stopped. The brick buildings and autumn trees spun.

It was the same drowning sensation I'd experienced in the final days that I practiced law. I gasped as if the air was thin and moved to the side of the road, just as I had when panic forced me to maneuver my car to a highway berm. I was back in the dirt of New Mexico, tears streaming down my face, plotting my demise.

Running was like everything else. I would fail. Time to lie down and curl into a ball.

"I'm going to pass out," I mumbled and bent over to bring the blood back to my head.

Julie's social-work skills kicked in. "Feel your feet, Nita Sweeney," she said gently, as if I were a lost child or a frightened animal. "Look at the flags. Can you feel your arms? Now look at the sky." I cupped my hands over my mouth to regulate my carbon dioxide to oxygen ratio.

Tapping into my meditation training, I tried to let the idea of quitting pass like a cloud floating across the sky. These thoughts and body sensations would pass if I let them. After a few moments, Julie began a slow jog. I had mentally tied myself to her. When she moved, so did I.

***

Then I realized my second mistake. I hadn't eaten since the stadium. I gobbled an electrolyte gel with some water to restore my depleted glycogen levels. It also distracted me from the panic. As we crossed Third, my vision focused. By the corner of Fifth Avenue, my breathing calmed, and my head cleared. My panic forgotten, I gave a disc jockey playing "Oh Mickey you're so fine..." a fist pump. On a downhill, Julie said, "You're speeding up!" In a tenth of a mile, I'd flipped from depression to mania. "We're going maximum speed, Nita Sweeney. Maximum speed!"

Mike Marshall stood on the bridge beyond Olentangy River Road. We yelled, hugged, and agreed it was torturous to have to climb the long Fifth Avenue hill at mile twenty-four. When I'd driven the route, it hadn't looked like a hill at all. We plodded on. Julie looked strong, but the hill strained my heavy legs and my throat filled with tears. It was a hill, I tell you, a bloody hill. So much for the mental techniques I'd practiced on the long runs. So much for mania.

The street was potholed again, and again I bumped into Julie. She ignored it. By the time we turned onto Neil, my short spurt of mania long gone, I was sure I couldn't go another step. My mind rebelled against the tediousness. The beautiful Victorian homes, spectacular fall foliage, and fans weren't enough stimulation. I longed for sleep.

At mile twenty-five, somewhere near Hubbard, a woman dressed in a black MIT shirt jumped up and down and waved her arms. I stared, not recognizing my friend, Lisa. I'd forgotten she would be there. When her identity clicked, I hugged her. She asked how I was. "In pain," I growled. "I'll run in with you," she said and continued chatting. This far into the race, I wanted to crawl into my little mental world, focus on form, or sing songs in my head the way I had when our group fell silent in the final miles of our Saturday runs. Lisa's cheerful conversation popped me out of my protective bubble. Julie told Lisa she was grateful for the distraction. Only then did I realize that Julie and I hadn't spoken for more than half a mile. Julie listened to Lisa while I sang "Jingle Bell Rock" in my head.

"You're so close," Lisa repeated. The mile markers and the numbers on my watch were a blur. I could not judge the distance.

Buttles sloped severely and, as we ran along Goodale Park, I kept sliding down the street. There was a little dip at the centerline and it didn't seem right. I told Lisa I needed to move off the line. I'm not sure there was actually a dip. I might have been hallucinating, but I thought the line made me trip. At the Goodale Park pond, I did not comprehend that we were less than three-quarters of a mile from the finish.

Back on Neil, Lisa had announced the last water station, but that hadn't registered either. I should have been elated. That meant we were close to done. But I was beyond sentiment. My body was numb, doing the impossible, and my mind rebelled. Lisa had enough emotion for the three of us, giggling while she talked as if joy bubbled from her mouth, while I despaired, certain we were destined to run forever.

My despondency continued as we approached mile twenty-six. Stacy, another running friend, grabbed my hand. "You're my hero." Her hand was warm and radiated love, but her kindness confused me. Holding her hand also made me run lopsided. "Thank you," I said. "I need my hand back now." She let go, and I left her.

"Mile twenty-six," Lisa said at the marker. The tall buildings ahead meant Nationwide Boulevard and the finish, must be near, but I was certain this agony would never end. As if in one last-ditch effort to stop me, an angry voice inside my head screamed, "Fuse! Fuse! Fuse!" and closed with the ultimate threat, "You're not going to survive this!" But I had Velcroed myself to Julie and wasn't letting go.

When I saw the red bricks of Nationwide Boulevard, sense memory kicked in and shut the negative voices down hard. We turned right and into view came the breathtaking vision of people milling about, empty bleachers, enormous loudspeakers, balloon arches, and a huge banner bearing the most glorious word I have ever seen: FINISH!

My mind clicked back on and joy filled my throat. "We did it!" I screamed. Hyperfocused, I found a higher gear and sprinted toward the line.

Then I remembered Julie. She had slowed to point out a sign saying, "Go Nita!" being held by my friend Krista and her son Tyler, the same Krista who, two and a half years before, had suggested I run races in the first place. Julie caught me as I blew kisses to Krista with tears streaming down my face. Throughout the race, I'd stemmed my emotions and conserved energy by being stoic, not high-fiving, not cheering much, and rarely yelling. Now, I hollered and wept as we careened toward that splendid line.

Julie fist-pumped and I threw my hands up in a victory sign as we crossed. Someone took a photo of us from behind, with me in my pink hat and Julie's ponytail swinging in the air. Volunteers put medals around our necks and gave us each a bottle of water.

Then I saw Ed, tears streaming down his face. He had snuck into the finish chute. I wrapped my arms around him and bawled. I didn't want to let go. I'd done it! I'd run a freaking marathon!

***

But I did let go of Ed. We thanked the volunteers, then Julie and I mounted the awful stairs at McFerson Commons Park to claim our food bags. I only wanted chocolate milk. My sister ran over and hugged me. Julie was mindful that some of our friends were still on the course, so we headed to the stands to watch them come in. Julie had her PR. We cheered Jennifer who, after all those miles, still looked as put-together as if she had merely jogged around the block. Julie went to talk to Jennifer, and I waited while Jim and Stephen came in. I was having trouble walking but wanted to greet them, so I waddled to the fence as best I could.

Stephen, introspective as usual, repeated how the marathon distance wasn't for him. He preferred the half. "It's good to learn these things," he said. A few days later, he and his wife were planning for the Chicago Marathon next fall. Jennifer and I had our photo taken in front of the MIT banner that bore all our names. "That's one and done!" she declared. The following season she would talk about not wanting her 26.2 sticker to get stale.

Like Stephen and Jennifer, I wasn't sure I wanted to run another full. When I asked Ed, he said, "It's waaay too soon to tell." That was the smartest answer, because by Tuesday I was thinking about what marathon to do next. The winner finished the full in 2:19:03 at a pace of 5:19 per mile. My time was 6:24:51 at a pace of 14:41. That was also the time on my Garmin, which was the first time it had been accurate since I owned it.

Eventually, Ed and I walked to the car. Getting in was excruciating. But oh how splendid it was to not have to run or even walk one more step. At home, I took an ice bath, then a hot shower. I put the medal around the dog's neck, but that just annoyed him. I also didn't take a nap.

***

That evening, our running group members wore race shirts and medals to Winking Lizard Tavern where we ate and reminisced. A group of faster runners welcomed Ed and me into their conversation. Ken, a tall, muscular man at the table, had qualified for the Boston Marathon. I don't know who was prouder, him of his "BQ" or me of my first "full." He and his fast friends treated me with respect. My legs hurt and I was exhausted. I could have stayed home, but I wanted to be with runners. Most people know the marathon is a huge feat, but until you've run one, you don't truly understand. We talked of highs and lows. I told them about tethering myself to Julie and how she talked me down from a panic attack. We laughed about our compulsiveness and high-fived our victories. The Deads also met late that afternoon, but I chose to be with MIT since I'd trained with them all year. I wound up exactly where I was supposed to be.

CHAPTER 26

Taking It In

On Monday, after the marathon, I tested the limits of my cooking skills to make packaged chicken soup and hot tea for Ed, who was home sick. His cold had worsened after he sat outside all day to watch me run. While he slept, I went for a massage. The masseuse asked about the race, and I broke my preferred silence by spending seventy minutes recounting the details.

Then I drove to FrontRunner. They were giving 26.2 stickers to anyone who brought in their medal. I remembered coveting the sticker on the back of that friend's car before I'd even run a 5k. I'd looked at the ground and not at his young face when I'd confided I wanted to earn one. He'd been so kind. Even though I was nearly his mother's age, he'd said, "Keep running and, in time, you will."

The FrontRunner staff congratulated me, but it was low-key. I imagined that most of the folks who work there and their clients run marathons much faster than I had. Still exhausted from the race and slipping into a post-race blah, I left sad.

At home, I cleaned the back car window and found the place of honor for the 26.2 sticker. I chose the upper right-hand corner, directly opposite the 13.1 sticker I'd earned the year before. I wanted to tell that friend whose sticker I'd seen so many years ago that I'd earned mine but had lost track of him. He'd been right. I kept running and eventually earned my own.

***

Tuesday, the post-race blues descended. Ed, who usually keeps his fears to himself, worried aloud that I might fall into a full-blown depressive episode. He'd seen me navigate prior post-race lulls, but the marathon was a mountain. The valley below could be an abyss.

Running held a prominent place in my mental health kit, as essential as medication and therapy. Running reduced the number of naps I took, increased my self-esteem, made me more accountable, prevented my psychiatrist from having to increase or change my medication, and likely kept me out of the hospital, but it hadn't cured me. The post-race depression struck hard. I invoked the usual post-race remedy and registered for the Columbus Turkey Trot. This gave me a new goal, but the blue mood lingered.

Ed, my friends, and my family had supported me on race day. They cheered at the start, on the course, at the stadium and at the finish with signs, shouts, and hugs. But their love hadn't stuck the way my sweat had. Now, sitting at home with the dog, I felt bereft. My medal and shirt weren't enough, either.

In just forty-eight hours, the race had become a blur. I'd tried to capture it in writing, but the memories were fading. People said, "You must feel great." I too had expected elation and a sense of accomplishment. Instead, I was sad, tired, grumpy, and sore. Despite having said I only wanted to finish, I'd hoped for a faster time. I'd also hoped the final miles wouldn't have been so hard.

Plus, I missed Mom, Dad, and Jamey. I knew they would have been proud, but their absence dug a hollowed-out place in my stomach. Uncle Johnny, the runner who preferred 10ks, sent a congratulatory email. I thanked him but lamented not experiencing the emotions people thought I should.

I hadn't made plans for the day, so I sat in my office and stared at Morgan. It miffed him that I'd raced without him. My shiny medal bored him. He'd run all those training miles with me. Where was his reward? I tried to explain. Before I finished, he was snoring.

If not for my aching legs, I might have thought the race had never happened. It was so typical of me to downplay an accomplishment. When someone congratulates me and I respond, "It was nothing," I mean "I didn't do enough." Never something to be proud of. By Tuesday afternoon, the compliments and hugs, the cheering and support, had slipped from memory. I needed to resurrect them, not for the external compliments, but to own it, to make that medal mine. I had run a marathon and needed to be proud of it.

***

If running taught me anything, it was how to turn things around. So many times, I had dreaded a workout, only for it to turn out splendid. So many days I had been convinced I would get lost. only to be thrilled by new scenery as I found my way. So many mornings I growled about rising at the butt-crack of dawn, then wound up laughing with my friends. This was no different. The doldrums wouldn't last, especially if I took action.

I pulled down the medal and picked up the shirt. Holding them empowered me. I changed into the shirt, put on the medal, and covered it with a fleece jacket.

First, I drove to the locally owned coffee shop where I am a regular. Colin, the owner and lead singer in the band Watershed, took time away from his orders to admire it. A few customers also wanted to see.

Next, I drove to a nearby grocery where some of my friends work. I showed them the medal and puffed up with pride. Each one congratulated and hugged me. Tim, the coffee roaster, teased, "How did you get in the front door with your head so big?" I laughed. "It nearly didn't fit!" Several customers congratulated me too. This day, unlike the day of the race, I was fully present and took in their words. My chest filled and the sadness dissipated. I was letting myself shine.

That night, I wore the medal to my recovery group. I let the hugs, compliments, and congratulations sink in. "Any semblance of humility I might have had is gone. Just GONE!" I said. A friend gave me a 26.2 mug and a pair of pink 26.2 socks. On the arch, they read, "I go all the way!" I let the warm sensations fill my body. I needed this delayed celebration. It extended the party the way it does when someone sends a late birthday card. My throat filled with tears. I was a marathoner!

***

The marathon reminded me of the three-day Ohio Bar Exam. The first day is essays, the second multiple choice, and the third more essays. Most people who fail do so during the last half of the third day. They give up, wind down, or burn out. For the test, people told me to pace myself, limiting the time and energy I spent on each question. I did so, hoping to be fully alert that third afternoon. It worked, and I passed. The same was true of the marathon. Those final miles beat me up but didn't defeat me.

In the days after the race, many people said, "What a life-changing experience!" In hindsight, crossing the finish line of a full marathon was more of a peak experience. I've had many. Finding out I'd passed the Bar Exam. The day Ed proposed. Our wedding day. Finishing my first 5k. All fabulous. But those aren't truly life-altering. What changes your life is the day-to-day stuff leading up to and following the events. The intense race moments are burned into memory. Catching Julie and Jennifer. Seeing the finish line. Throwing my arms around Ed. But that's not what changed me.

Those peaks resulted from training. Following the schedule unless there was a good reason not to, not just one day, but the entire season. Showing up over and over to lace my shoes and push out the door. Getting up at four thirty in the morning to run double-digit miles. Watching my body grow stronger and muscles develop under my skin, even as my mind told me it was impossible. When I'd begun to train, a naive part of me thought, "No big deal. Just put one foot in front of the other!" Ironically, that's how you do it. One foot in front of the other, mile after mile, over weeks and weeks. My life was altered by not being derailed.

When an email announced official race photos, I scanned them hungrily. There we were in the cold at the start. There we were at various mile markers. And thankfully, there we were at the finish.

I cheered out loud, waking the dog from a sound sleep, when I noticed I wasn't heel-striking. In some photos, my knees were too bent or I was hunched, but I was landing midfoot! My soreness after the race would have been worse if I'd been landing on my heels. ChiRunning, good form running, natural form running, the pose method, and focusing on form had worked. I wasn't aware during the race. I was just trying not to die. But the photos were proof. I had changed my form.

I scrolled through again, trying to choose a few, then laughed and bought the whole set. The commemorative CD would serve as evidence when I forgot I'd done it. There it was in color. Me in Bexley not heel-striking. Me in German Village smiling. Me at Ohio Stadium laughing. Me on Neil Avenue grimacing. Me running the marathon my mind told me I never could.

***

In the weeks after the race, my hip and knees hurt, but the years of training had transformed the aches and pains I'd felt more than two years before. My huge swollen ankle had morphed into minor sensations in my knee and hip. Continuing to move regardless of the pain had made the difference. I hadn't ignored the pain, but wouldn't give in either. I didn't listen to the surgeon who wanted to cut me open or my primary care physician who said my running days were numbered. Instead, I looked for solutions: Egoscue, stretching, learning to run differently, and transitioning to different shoes. The desire to continue running for the rest of my life made me willing to try nearly anything.

Plenty of people think I'm obsessed or addicted. Given the improvement in my mental health, I'll claim it as healthy. Others think I'm ruining by body. "Your knees and joints will wear out. A doctor will tell you to quit." Too late! A doctor already told me to quit. I don't think I'm naive or stupid. I just need to stick with people who "get" running.

Many people do everything I did and still get injured. I count myself lucky, but the jury is still out on me as a test subject. The Deads were the first ones I heard say that each of us is "an experiment of one." Others have confirmed it. If I'm still running twenty years from now, I'll get on my soapbox. Until then, I'll shut my mouth and be grateful.

***

Shortly after the marathon, I had my teeth cleaned. The dental hygienist runs, mostly chasing her children. She asked about the marathon and for advice about aches and pains. I shared about Egoscue, running form, and shoes. We talked about rest days, stretching, and training plans. Watching her nod reminded me I knew a thing or two. I am a real runner.

By this time, I believed so strongly in the healing power of running that I would talk about my adventure to anyone. I'd gone from a woman who found it difficult to leave her house to one who regularly took part in enormous events with total strangers. Time alone on the trail or the streets had become a meditation, a time for reflection, and a path of insight. Running with a group taught me I could be social without being overwhelmed. Training helped me to show up regardless of how I felt, even if it meant getting up at hours I fondly referred to as "the middle of the night." Facing my fears gave me a sense of self-esteem I'd often lacked. My days slouched alone on the sofa jealously reading social media posts about my friend's accomplishments were over. I joined their ranks and had the strong legs to show for it. Because of the positive way running had transformed by body and mind, I eagerly shared my joy.

***

The Wednesday after the race, the dog and I took our first post-race run. The lady walker who wears a dress and whose keeshond always barks was out, with her cat following close behind. Workers in Donna Ravine continued renovating the sewers. Jim, the mail carrier, gave Morgan his biscuit, and the Chihuahuas bounced in their bay window like tiny cheerleaders. Rain had given way to sunshine, so the neighborhood lawns were more gorgeously green than usual. I even enjoyed running up Fairlington Hill, which I sometimes dread. Slow. Easy. As we jogged down the street, tears choked my throat. I'd run a marathon!

My thoughts turned to my training. While I'd completed the official MIT sixteen-week full marathon training schedule, my real training had begun in March 2010, when I timidly left my house, dressed in cotton, wearing heavy trail shoes, carrying a kitchen timer, and tugging the dog out the door for a sixty-second jog. I remembered my high school friend Kim's posts and the emails from my London friend, Fiona, about buying her first pair of "trainers." I thought of all the times Wendy the ultramarathoner had talked about running. I recalled running in my early thirties, even though my motives were unhealthy and not what I want them to be today. My training for a full marathon had taken every decade.

And I thought of the mental training. I'd drawn on endless hours of writing practice and meditation, plus thousands of recovery meetings. Over twenty years, I'd learned to do what was in front of me and throw myself into something despite the voices in my head. Keep your hand moving. Continue under all circumstances. Don't be afraid to make mistakes or look foolish. Suit up and show up. Stay in the present. Don't be tossed away. These key lessons prepared me to finish both the training and the race.

I also remembered the amazing running community. Weekend long runs with the running group had been fun and important. My heart filled with gratitude for MIT and my running friends, the water on the trail, the change of scenery, and the great conversations.

And I thought fondly of Ed, my rock, who cheered me on and kept our home together as I spent hours on the streets and trails. I wondered how I'd gotten so lucky.

Still, as the dog and I ran that morning, a naked truth stood out. The lion's share of training had been just like this run: an ordinary weekday run through our neighborhood, me, the dog, the watch, and the road. Morgan and I had run down this very street in hot, humid weather when I carried two water bottles for me and a third for him. We'd run in falling snow and pouring rain, stopping only for me to eat a gel and him a ziplock bag of kibble. And while we'd both hated and loved those beagles and Chihuahuas, there'd been no one in the neighborhood making us run and no fanfare. No Coach Julie to Velcro myself to. No LeDawn to sherpa our stuff. No Ed or Amy or anyone else cheering. No bands, no expo, no medal. No Jeff, the Tall Guy, no Kelley or Stephen, no post-run chocolate milk or bagels.

Here in the neighborhood, on regular days like this, we had done it by ourselves, one foot in front of the other.

It really was that simple. Not easy, but not complicated. It was like any other goal—going back to school or moving across the country. You bring dreams to fruition by doing the work in front of you. You put in the effort and, most of the time, get results. If I, an overweight fifty-year-old with chronic depression, manic episodes, anxiety, hypochondria, and a wonky ankle could do it, anyone could.

My feet were light, my stride easy, and my foot turnover quick. It felt like flying, just like in my dreams!

Epilogue

Months passed. The memory of running the marathon began to seem like a dream. Part of me wanted to train for a second full. Another part feared the first marathon had been a fluke.

On a humid August morning, ten months after the race, Mr. Dawg and I once again trotted through the neighborhood. "Well?" I asked, thinking of another full. He nodded or perhaps shook a bug off his ear. That night at dinner, I asked Ed. At first, he laughed. "You forgot how hard it was." But he saw my earnestness, put his hand over mine, and said, "I know you can do it again."

A few days later, Julie texted that the 2013 Columbus Marathon was on record pace to sell out. I looked at Morgan, who lay at my feet. "Whaddya think, Pink?" His ears perked up and his eyes gleamed. When he cocked his head, I went online and signed up.

Conclusion and Resources

As it turns out, running my first marathon was NOT a fluke. I ran that second marathon and a third several years later. And remember those books I couldn't finish writing? Well, you're holding my pride and joy. I'll repeat what I said in the "Author's Note" at the beginning of this book: "Your mileage may vary" (YMMV). I learned what works for me. I do not know what will work for you. You must create your own story. But here are some resources I find helpful.

Writing Books

Bestselling author Natalie Goldberg's *Writing Down the Bones* put me on a solid path. Other writing books that will never leave my bookshelf include *Bird by Bird* by Annie LaMott, *The Writing Life* by Annie Dillard, *If You Want to Write* by Brenda Ueland, and *The Situation and the Story* by Vivian Gornick. But nothing beats close reading with an eye to how the writer created the story. There you will find your own "teachers."

Meditation Books

Mindfulness in Plain English by Bhante Gunaratana remains my favorite because it opens by answering the question, "Why bother?" Other texts I return to are *Zen in the Art of Archery* by Eugen Herrigel, *One Bird, One Stone* by Sean Murphy, *Wherever You Go, There You Are* by Jon Kabat-Zinn, *Everyday Zen* by Charlotte Joko Beck, and *The Science of Enlightenment* by Shinzen Young. Shinzen.org also has a series of downloadable recordings. In the "old days," Ed and I owned more than a hundred cassette tapes of Shinzen lectures. I listened in my car. It was a sad day when I bought a car without a cassette player.

Running Books

If you haven't read *Born to Run* by Christopher McDougall, stop right now and buy it. Buy the audio version. You won't want it to end.

Other books I found helpful or inspiring were *ChiRunning* by Danny Dreyer, *Unbroken* by Laura Hillenbrand, *Once a Runner* by John L. Parker Jr. (all his books are fabulous, including his *Heart Rate Training for the Compleat Idiot*), Natural Running by Danny Abshire, *The Pose Method of Running* by Nicholas Romanov, and *The Non-Runner's Marathon Trainer* by David A. Whitsett, Forrest Allen Dolgener, and Tanjala Mabon Kole. And *Running is My Therapy* by Scott Douglas puts science behind my experience. Having a running book going makes me want to get out there!

One Good Earbud

I don't run with earbuds, even on trails. Remember how Morgan and I almost got hit by a truck near that landscaper when I couldn't hear the truck coming, even with only one earbud in? That's why. But when I did wear them, I wore One Good Earbud. They are literally that. One earbud. Please don't get killed.

Running Movies

Watching a movie about running, especially in the company of other runners, is so inspiring. My favorites include *Spirit of the Marathon*, *Chariots of Fire*, *Running on the Sun*, *My Run*, and *The Long Run*, but there are many great ones.

Diet

YMMV is most true here. The only common factor when it comes to diet is that you can't outrun your mouth. Ed and I used to joke about belonging to the "diet of the month club" because we'd try nearly any diet that came down the pike. For most of the time period covered in the book, I followed the Slow Carb Diet from Tim Ferriss' book *The Four-Hour Body* (recommended to me by my ultrarunner friend and neighbor, Luke Tuttle). I lost weight and kept it off for several years, until I couldn't stand to see one more bean. Now, I follow the principles in *On Eating* by Susie Orbach. While I gained back some weight, I feel more mindful and calm around food.

Good Form Running

If a running store near you holds a "GFR" class offered by New Balance, take it. There are also online resources. I had a foundation of ChiRunning and had read a lot about form before I took a class, but GFR was a fabulous crash course in form and solidified what I already knew.

Egoscue Method and Active Isolated Stretching

Ed told me about Egoscue years ago and it was life-changing. I no longer spend weeks on the sofa with back pain. I still do several "e-cises" daily, especially the "gravity drop" and the "static back press." Luke Tuttle (the ultramarathoner mentioned above) turned me on to "AIS." I do it daily too. Egoscue works on cold muscles because "e-cises" are postures and movements, not stretches. And Active Isolated Stretching is, well, not static! Research shows that static stretching can strain cold muscles.

Mapping Routes, Logging Your Runs, and Tracking Your Gear

When I began this journey, MapMyRun was the thing. I still use it, but I'm old. Now Strava is the thing. There will be a new thing after that. Garmin Connect has been a constant. It's not terribly helpful with mapping a route, but will track your data exquisitely. I now use all three, but MapMyRun feels like home.

Training Plans

Morgan and I began our training following the "Couch to 5k" program from coolrunnning.com. At the time, the plan was on their website. Now, there is an app. Once I joined Marathoner in Training, they provided the training plan. It is similar to those offered online by Hal Higdon. Recently, I have begun to follow the plans offered by Olympian Jeff Galloway. Compare plans and find your fit.

A Watch

I started with a kitchen timer. It was ridiculous, but it worked for me! Then I moved to a Timex Ironman, and now I'm on my third

Garmin Forerunner. I like data, bells, and whistles. I like to know my heart rate and pace and intervals and cadence and vertical oscillation and vertical ratio (whatever that is). I don't need most of it, and don't understand all of it, but I like it! Some people run without a watch. I am not one of those people.

Metronome

I love my clip-on Seiko DM51. It made figuring out and increasing my cadence much simpler. Now, some watches have a built-in metronome.

Shoes

Go to a good running store like Fleet Feet and let them fit you. Trust them when they say you need a much larger size than you normally wear. Your feet will swell when you run. And if the shoes make any noise or rub anywhere on your first run, take them back right away. You will not get used to them and the last thing you need is a blister or a stress fracture from wearing the wrong shoes. But also take with a grain of salt what the sales person may say about pronation or supination or any other nation. Try what is recommended, but always trust yourself. Learn to feel your body. I love my Newtons.

What to Wear

In central Ohio, it can be fifty-two degrees on Tuesday and twenty-eight with a "feels like" seven degrees rating on Saturday. Figuring out what to wear on a run is akin to rocket science. I love both the "What to Wear" tool from *Runner's World* and the dressmyrun.com website. I'm usually cold, so I add a layer. My warm-blooded friends leave off a layer. Again, trial and error is your friend, but never wear cotton!

Long-Run Fodder

Learn jokes or gather topics to discuss with your running group or ponder on long runs. When I practiced law, I "collected" lawyer jokes, so I could say the punch line before the person telling the joke finished. Now, much to the distress of my pace group mates,

I tell lawyer jokes on long runs. Subscribe to the "Dumb Runner" newsletter. Mark Remy, a former *Runner's World* columnist, is hilarious. His weekly newsletter includes topics to discuss on your long run. More than once they've been a life-saver.

Gels and Beans and Snacks

If I'm running more than four miles, I take something to eat. Some of the Dead Runners Society folks swear they never take a gel unless they're running ten miles. I'm not that hard-core—or that fast! Experts say runners need to replenish glycogen stores. I take a Clif Shot every forty-five minutes and chase it with a handful of Brazil nuts and Marcona almonds (the kind without skins). On runs longer than ten miles, I need "real" food. Peanut butter and jelly sandwiches proved to be too messy. Now I eat peanut butter crackers in addition to the gels and nuts. Running nutrition is another serious YMMV area. Try things for yourself, but please experiment only on your training runs, so you're not in distress come race day.

Sports Drinks

Some of my "Dead" friends run marathons drinking only water. I'm not sure when Gatorade first appeared on race courses, but it wasn't always there. Still, I like to have the option on longer runs, or if the weather is especially warm or especially cold. Both extremes will dehydrate and deplete electrolytes. I made homemade "Gatorade" for a while but grew bored. Now I use Skratch Labs electrolyte drink powder. This is another developing area. A new thing will come along and the Boston winner will be drinking it. You might as well try that. It might be exactly what you need.

Community

Although I'm an "off-the-scale" introvert, finding like-minded people is vital. First the Penguins and the Dead Runners Society, and then Marathoner in Training through Fleet Feet Sports Columbus, provided a running family. In writing, I found other writers while attending Natalie Goldberg's writing workshops. I also participate in National Novel Writing Month (nanowrimo.org) every November and belong to several central Ohio writing clubs. A meditation community is called a "sangha." Ed and I have attended meditation groups and retreats of many types and found community there. If you can't find the type of group you need, attend a class or a meetup, and make your own!

The Bottom Line

Try something. Anything. Orange Theory or Parkour or yoga with goats. Haiku or fables or portrait memoir. Zen or Tibetan or Vipassana. For me, any small action—breaking a sweat, writing a paragraph, sitting for five minutes—makes a huge difference. I hope it will for you, as well.

Acknowledgments

Writing is a team sport. Growing a book requires the love, care, expertise, and support of a tribe. If we've ever met, you helped make this book happen.

Infinite gratitude to my long-time teacher, Natalie Goldberg, for giving me writing practice. Everything springs from that.

No words can express my appreciation for Tania Casselle and Sean Murphy. Your teaching, editing, coaching, and moral support shaped the book, taught me the business of writing, and kept me sane.

Thanks to the wrimos of National Novel Writing Month for allowing me to rebel not once, not twice, not three times, but four times, as I wrestled with this book. Thanks for all the stickers!

Pat Snyder, Mitsy Andrews, Shirley Hyatt, Wendy Drake, Jill Blixt, Marcia Dahlinghaus, and Kae Denino each deserve a standing ovation for slogging through early drafts and pointing out the potential.

Thanks to my "Words in the World" classmates Victoria Hubbell, Mag Dimond, Sherry Hardage, Stephanie McKinney, Jan Smith, and the late Martha McMullen for honesty, wisdom, and laughter.

And much love and gratitude to my own students across the decades for teaching me what I need to learn.

Love and hugs to the women of Writeth-On: Marie Radanovich, Pat Snyder, Mitsy Andrews, Shirley Hyatt, Lora Fish, Joy Schroeder, Cheryl Peterson, Krista Hilton, Alison Hazelbaker, Sally Stamper, Martha Crone, Sammi Soutar, Marilyn Peters, Laura Staley, Faith Van Horn, and all the "substitutes," for listening, nodding, smiling, laughing, rolling your eyes, and giving me space. And thanks to our incredible Metroparks for saving the trees, deer, and wild turkeys so we can write in your special venue.

While rejection is never fun, I appreciate the agents, editors, and contest judges who took the time to offer feedback and encouragement.

Many thanks to Colin Gawel of Colin's Coffee for encouraging me to hog the table by the door for hours on end. And a shout-out to Tim Blair and the entire staff at Kingsdale Market District for cheering me and feeding me and letting me hang out.

Without the runners, this book would have remained a dream. Thank you to every runner who waved, nodded, or high-fived. Special thanks to Marathoner in Training, Jeff Henderson, Tim Flahaven, Lucky 13s, 13 R/W, 14 R/W, Yep It's Just Us Runners, Dead Runners Society, Penguins, Still I Run, Half Fanatics, 50 States Half Marathon Club, and 100 Half Marathons Club, and anyone with whom I've ever shared the pavement. You provide the structure to keep me and my fellow road warriors moving. And extra special thanks with sprinkles on top to Kim Watton for introducing me to "Couch to 5k," Fiona Thompson for writing about "trainers," and Julie DeBord for talking me down time and again.

Much appreciation to Scott Edelstein for his wisdom and calm demeanor. Your guidance is invaluable.

Words fail to capture my gratitude for Brenda Knight and the experts at Mango Publishing. Thank you for believing in me and this project and showing me the ropes. I continue to learn and grow under your care.

A deep bow to the church-basement, folding-chair, coffee-pot people who help me stay on the path.

Amy Ax, my sweet sister, you deserve my undying loyalty for your steadfast support and willingness to listen to me whine when it is you who bears the real burden. To the rest of my family, I always knew you had my back. Thank you.

I've had the great fortune to be loved by many dogs, but none so incredible as Morgan, who remained my deep teacher to the end of his days. Thanks also to Scarlet, for helping us smile again after Morgan died.

But my eternal devotion goes to Ed Sweeney, the love of my life, who saves me over and over, day after day. Thank you for everything, always. My love for you knows no bounds. Tap. Tap. Tap.

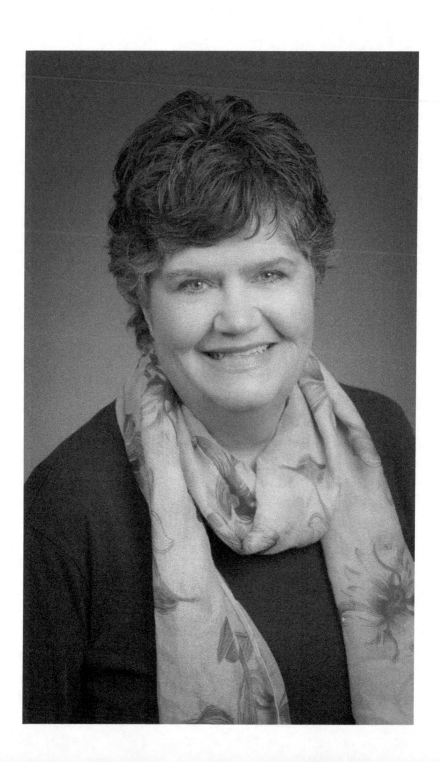

About the Author

Nita Sweeney's articles, essays, and poems have appeared in *Buddhist America, Dog World, Dog Fancy, Writer's Journal, Country Living, Pitkin Review, Spring Street, The Taos News, WNBA-SF blog,* and other newspapers and newsletters. She writes a blog, *Bum Glue,* and publishes a monthly email, the *Write Now Newsletter.*

She has been featured on Health.com, Healthline.com, Livestrong.com, and Medium.com, as well as in *bp Magazine* and on the *Word Carver* and *My Brain on Endorphins* podcasts. Nita was nominated for the Ohio Arts Council Governor's Award. Her poem "Memorial" won the Dublin Arts Council's Poet's Choice Award and her memoir, *Depression Hates a Moving Target: How Running with My Dog Brought Me Back from the Brink* (formerly titled *Twenty-Six Point Freaking Two*) was short-listed for the William Faulkner–William Wisdom Creative Writing Competition Award.

Nita earned a journalism degree from the E. W. Scripps School of Journalism at Ohio University, a law degree from the Ohio State University, and a Master of Fine Arts degree in Creative Writing from Goddard College. For ten years, she studied with and assisted bestselling author Natalie Goldberg (*Writing Down the Bones*) at week-long writing workshops, teaching the "rules of writing practice" and leading participants in sitting and walking meditation. Goldberg authorized Nita to teach "writing practice," and Nita has taught for nearly twenty years.

When she's not writing and teaching, Nita runs. She has completed three full marathons, twenty-six half marathons (in eighteen states), and more than sixty shorter races. Nita lives in central Ohio with her husband and biggest fan, Ed, and her yellow Labrador running partner, Scarlet the #ninetyninepercentgooddog.

For more information or to subscribe to Nita's newsletter, please visit nitasweeney.com.

CPSIA information can be obtained
at www.ICGtesting.com
Printed in the USA
BVHW031618120719
553303BV00001B/1/P

9 781642 500134